Revitalize Your Hormones

Dr. Dale's 7 Steps to a Happier,
Healthier, and Sexier You

Theresa Dale, N.D., C.C.N., Ph.D

D0062286

WILEY

John Wiley & Sons, Inc.

Published by John Wiley & Sons, Inc., Hoboken, New Jersey
Published simultaneously in Canada

Design and composition by Navta Associates, Inc.

For general information about our other products and services, please contact our Customer Care Department within the United States at (800) 762-2974, outside the United States at (317) 572-3993 or fax (317) 572-4002.

Wiley also publishes its books in a variety of electronic formats. Some content that appears in print may not be available in electronic books. For more information about Wiley products, visit our web site at www.wiley.com.

Library of Congress Cataloging-in-Publication Data:

Dale, Theresa.
    Revitalize your hormones : Dr. Dale's 7 steps to a happier, healthier, and sexier you / Theresa Dale.
        p. cm.
    Includes bibliographical references and index.
    ISBN-10 0-471-65555-4 (paper)
    ISBN-13 978-0-471-65555-8 (paper)
    1. Middle aged women—Health and hygiene. 2. Middle aged women—Nutrition. 3. Menopause—Alternative treatment. 4. Perimenopause—Alternative treatment. 5. Endocrine gynecology. 6. Rejuvenation. 7. Hormones. I. Title.
    RA778.D236 2005
    618.1'7506—dc22

                                                                                        2004027107

Printed in the United States of America

10 9 8 7 6 5 4 3

Contents

Foreword

The revolutionary premise of *Revitalize Your Hormones: Dr. Dale's 7 Steps to a Happier, Healthier, and Sexier You* is that you can balance your hormones naturally, without using expensive and risky drugs, and that hormone revitalization will make you feel and look your best ever. Unlike other books on women's health and hormones, *Revitalize Your Hormones* provides evidence-based, proven-effective strategies for hormone vitalization. These methods are far superior to hormone replacement therapy (HRT), which carries well-documented, life-threatening risks.

Dr. Dale's program has already balanced the hormones of almost three thousand women, and she has the hormone saliva tests to prove it. The program in *Revitalize Your Hormones* is revelatory news for the approximately 38 million female baby boomers who seek to take control of their hormones and enjoy their prime years without drugs or synthetic bio-identical hormones.

This last point is especially vital to women who are wondering about their hormone health options. Even natural hormones such as those in the progesterone cream Pro-Gest have been found in some studies to raise progesterone levels to toxically high levels, thus exposing users to the same elevated disease risks faced by women taking conventional drug HRT. I would like to stress that with Dr. Dale's safe and effective program, there are zero health risks and only potential health benefits.

Invoking the power of the endocrine system and the body's innate ability to continue making hormones after menopause, Dr. Dale's program involves detoxification, organic nutrition, stress management, emotional self-management, exercise, and homeopathy to reeducate the body to produce hormones in appropriate amounts. Unlike conventional or bio-identical hormone replacement therapy,

Dr. Dale's program allows women to tap their inborn healing potential and explore their emotional terrain in order to balance hormones in the long term.

In Dr. Dale's practice, your mind/body is your friend, and this book shows you how to care for your lifelong friend with empowering lifestyle changes and natural remedies. Using safe, nontoxic, and effective homeopathy, the second-most widely used system of medicine in the world, Dr. Dale provides remedies for women's health conditions and common medical problems.

This book offers great value to the consumer. Its pages contain breakthrough and possibly life-saving health information, much of which is published here for the first time. Action plans at the end of each chapter remind readers of the steps they must take to make progress toward balancing their hormones. Exercise suggestions, meditation guidelines, nutrition regimens, and delicious recipes also help support hormone health along the way. The Resource Guide at the end of the book is a veritable encyclopedia of products for natural living. This is yet another way that *Revitalize Your Hormones* can help you improve your quality of life and your health, now and in the long term.

It is a pleasure to recommend *Revitalize Your Hormones* to you and to health-care professionals who seek a safe and effective alternative to the perils of all forms of HRT. I have known Dr. Dale for years and am familiar with her many successes in treating hormone imbalances with natural remedies. Besides being a naturopath, she is also a certified clinical nutritionist, whose talent for nutritional healing is highly developed, as you will see in chapter 4. I would also like you to know that Dr. Dale is such a highly valued colleague that I am a faculty member at her California state-approved college, the California College of Natural Medicine.

The ability of Dr. Dale's program to revitalize and balance hormones in women who have had complete hysterectomies is one of the major natural healing advances of this century; it holds the potential to help millions of women stay strong and sexy without using drugs that have undesirable side effects and that elevate disease risk.

Contrary to popular belief, radiant health and positive aging are your birthright. Dr. Dale's natural healing protocol gives you all the tools you need to manage your health destiny for maximum mind-body balance and well-being. All you have to do is use them to care for yourself. Remember, you know your body better than anyone else does, and with Dr. Dale's program, you have the power to reeducate your body to make hormones in appropriate amounts, now and for the rest of your life.

Earl Mindell, Ph.D, R.Ph.

Acknowledgments

My sincere gratitude to Kyle Roderick, whose assistance in writing, structure, and editorial services helped to communicate my voice and commitment to readers; John Higley, who provided creative graphics services; Malcolm Riley, for his positive support and inspiration; and my patients, for the privilege of assisting them in their evolution.

Introduction

For twenty years, I have helped patients to correct hormonal imbalances through the use of homeopathic remedies and the many healing strategies detailed in this book. My program expanded and evolved when I began to experience perimenopausal ups and downs that echoed my mother's symptoms. At that point, I realized what an important role genetics plays in the change of life, and I discovered how simply and easily symptoms can be remedied.

My own health, along with my desire to provide women with nontoxic and natural hormone revitalization strategies, compelled me to create a 7-Step Program in 1999. Since then, I've refined and perfected the program to make it as effective and user-friendly as possible.

At the core of my program are these seven principles:

- understand the dangers of all forms of hormone replacement therapy (HRT)
- get to know your hormones and why they go out of balance
- detoxify your body
- follow dietary guidelines for hormone rejuvenation
- learn and practice stress-management techniques
- develop emotional awareness so that emotions are easily managed
- use homeopathy to reeducate the body to make hormones in appropriate amounts

In addition, monitor your newfound health by taking notes on your progress and cook with hormone-balancing, healthful recipes, to reinforce your success on the program.

Since I developed and started to practice my program, I have readjusted my hormonal levels and rejuvenated my body to the point where I feel wonderfully vibrant. I have shared this program with hundreds of physicians, osteopaths, and chiropractors around the world, as well as with women in my private practice. Hundreds of health-care professionals, including physicians, consult with me because they find conventional hormone replacement therapy (HRT) and so-called natural hormone replacement therapies to be variously ineffective, irritating, and toxic.

In fact, many health-care providers whom I work with, including physicians, report that they tried my program because they realized that there had to be a safer and better way to balance hormones, without taking synthetic or compounded natural ones—which, despite their misleading name, are synthesized in a laboratory.

This book is the first guide for women that explores the complexities of their hormone health and offers easy, effective action plans, all without drugs or surgery. You will learn how to balance hormone levels, improve your health, and enhance your quality of life. As you'll discover, my system of balancing hormones involves reassessing and changing your lifestyle and exercise habits to promote optimum health, by the use of safe, gentle homeopathic formulas. My hormone revitalization program is based upon the premise that our bodies are natural, exquisitely powerful, and unique systems that were designed to maintain a balance through individualized care, which encompasses nutrition, meditation, and yoga.

I would like to help every woman who reads this book discover the unique truths about her body. Even if you have never studied health, nutrition, or medicine, by the time you finish this book, you will know more about your body than ever before, and you'll have the tools to heal yourself. The action plans in the first seven chapters give you information to help you connect the dots between your symptoms, your moods, your lifestyle, and nutrition, as well as natural remedies to revitalize your mind/body/hormones.

The medical establishment's approach to balancing hormones fails to embrace the concept of the body as a natural living system that is capable of self-repair. Rather, its treatment regimens are based on the premise that we need to look outside our bodies for hormone help via one-size-fits-all drugs.

Studies have shown that using hormones topically or orally causes the body to shut down production of its own natural hormones and creates a dependency that ages every organ and bodily system. It's also been scientifically proved that orally or topically used hormones can elevate existing hormone levels to toxically high amounts. This overload then taxes the adrenal glands, triggering the release of abnormal levels of the stress hormone cortisol, which makes women feel chronically exhausted and stressed and causes other uncomfortable symptoms.

My drug- and hormone-free program offers a safe, nontoxic, hormone-revitalizing alternative. Positive and graceful aging is your birthright, whereas conventional and natural hormone replacement therapy toxically burdens the entire body, including the liver, the kidneys, and the circulatory and immune systems.

The healing techniques that I learned as a traditional naturopath never include the use of drugs or surgery. Naturopathy is a European medical practice that uses homeopathic medicine, herbs, food, and other natural substances to bring the body into healthy balance by stimulating its innate immune defenses, without the use of drugs. In Europe, naturopathy is a revered medical tradition that is highly advanced and widely practiced. I chose to study in Germany and the United States, where the most progressive research on natural healing is done. After I cured myself of a uterine tumor (I am still not sure whether the tumor was fibroid or cancerous) with natural remedies at age twenty-two, my path became clear. I decided to specialize in natural hormone rejuvenation and to devote myself to helping humanity by using all of the knowledge I had acquired through years of study.

I received a degree as a naturopathic doctor from Clayton University in St. Louis, Missouri. Then I received board certification as a naturopathic doctor through the American Naturopathic Medical Association, licensed in Washington, D.C. I also studied nutrition extensively and achieved the designation certified clinical nutritionist with certification from the International and American Association of Applied Clinical Nutritionists.

After working with degenerative disease in private practice for more than a decade, I decided to focus my attention on natural hormone rejuvenation. My passion is to help humanity from my heart— and with all the knowledge I had acquired through years of study.

More than ten years ago, I founded the California College of Natural Medicine in Santa Barbara and Santa Cruz, California. There I teach several courses (which I created), including those for Holistic Health Practitioners, Advanced Holistic Health Practitioners, and

NeuroPhysical Reprogramming (NPR). I also created the curriculum for a program called Homeopathic Endocrinology Training, which involves balancing hormones with homeopathic remedies.

As you may know, homeopathy is a therapeutic system of medicine that is based on the principle of similars—like cures like. This means that a substance that may cause certain symptoms in a healthy person can also cure similar symptoms in an unhealthy person. Created and codified two hundred years ago by the German physician Samuel Hahnemann, homeopathy is recognized by the World Health Organization (WHO) as a therapeutic system and is approved by the FDA. Vast numbers of people, from Queen Elizabeth and the royal family of England to record-setting Olympic gold medalists like the Austrian skier Hermann Maier, use homeopathic remedies.

Homeopathy stimulates the body's innate defense and immune processes. You will learn the ABCs of this fascinating, effective, and relatively inexpensive form of healing in chapter 7. Homeopathic medicines are derived from a variety of plants, animal substances, and minerals. What makes them so powerful is that a specific remedy contains only a minute amount of any given ingredient (similar to, but significantly less than, that in a vaccination), which awakens the power of the body's immune system. This minute amount of an ingredient is so small that it is likened to a "memory" of the ingredient.

Along with being a state-approved director and an instructor at the California College of Natural Medicine, I am a passionate researcher and an inventor of holistic therapies and treatment methods. I created a highly accurate hormone saliva test that is used by hundreds of physicians, chiropractors, and other health-care providers. The test is based on the Chinese Five Element Theory, which you will learn about in chapter 2.

My research includes more than two thousand before-and-after medical saliva test results on doctors' patients, which prove that my hormone revitalization program has a 95 percent success rate with women, even with women who have had complete hysterectomies. Success means that the patient feels better and the hormone levels are balanced within a healthy, normal range. When the results of my program were reported, first in *Alternative Medicine* magazine and then at the American Naturopathic Medical Association's convention, followed by an article in *Spa* magazine, my office was inundated with phone calls from women urgently requesting assistance from me and my affiliate doctors.

My salivary testing research and twenty years of experience as a naturopathic doctor enabled me to develop the action plans and healing methods in this book. As a result, you now have your own healing tool kit, and you can start to balance your hormones without a saliva test. Furthermore, the program in this book is a medically proven alternative to so-called natural or bio-identical hormone replacement therapy. This has been shown in some studies to raise hormones to toxically high levels, which can be problematic for your health.

I am heartened by the fact that hundreds of licensed health-care providers, including ob/gyns, osteopaths, chiropractors, and so on, have attended my professionals' presentations, or they consult with me on homeopathic hormone-balancing regimens for their patients. The utilization of my program by various types of health-care professionals proves that the old medical model for treating hormone imbalance is beginning to dissolve. I invite you to surf the waves of this change by taking control of your hormones and maximizing your health.

This book will empower you to balance your hormones and enjoy optimum health, energy, sex drive, and happiness—all of which are your birthright. Before we begin our journey, let us take a deep breath to relax our minds and bodies. Breathe deeply, in through your nose, for six seconds or more, so that your chest expands and your lungs fill up with fresh air. Hold the breath for five seconds; now slowly exhale for six seconds, through your mouth, making sure to expel every last ounce of air. Congratulations! You have just learned one of the most effective stress-management techniques of all time. Now, let's begin the journey to a happier, healthier, and sexier you!

Part One

What You Need to Know about Your Body and Hormones

Step 1

Understanding the Dangers of Hormone Replacement Therapy

After finishing a lecture recently, I was approached by Sarah, an office manager with a hectic schedule who said that she was desperately seeking relief from hot flashes and perimenopausal symptoms. Sarah was prepared to try anything to get relief. As she listed the various hormone combinations her doctor had prescribed, I empathized how Sarah's story typified so many women's perimenopausal predicaments.

Sarah had tried conventional hormone replacement therapy (HRT) (drugs made from a combination of synthetic estrogen and synthetic progesterone, also known as progestin). She had also taken so-called natural or bio-identical HRT (pills, liquids, patches, or skin creams containing hormones that are synthesized in the laboratory and derived from either wild yam or soy). Even the so-called natural, bio-identical HRT caused her symptoms to intensify.

Doubts about the safety of taking so many chemicals over the years compounded Sarah's uneasiness. Like many other women whom I speak to, Sarah had become increasingly concerned that taking HRT chemicals might negatively affect her health.

Sarah's story is fairly typical. From my private practice, I know that women feel frustrated and often desperate about their hormone health options, and they worry about the dangers involved in taking conventional or natural HRT. I know how depressed you can get when you believe that you lack a safe alternative to HRT and you feel stuck in an unhealthful lifestyle. Nonetheless, you can relax now, because I am going to tell you about natural, effective choices that will help you feel healthier, sexier, and stronger.

Contrary to what the media and your doctor may lead you to believe, your body has the ability to produce the hormones it needs for as long as you are alive. For example, when the ovaries shut down after menopause, the adrenal glands continue producing progesterone and other hormones. Studies show that a healthy endocrine system is essential to making hormones in appropriate amounts throughout life. While chapters 3 through 7 detail numerous effective endocrine-support strategies, part 3 provides recipes and pantry and food guidelines that you can use to nourish your body and mind for the rest of your life.

Another key point: hormone health depends not on age or where you are on the perimenopausal or postmenopausal spectrum. It depends on a complex of factors, such as the air that you breathe; the water you drink; the quality of your diet, sleep, and exercise; the relative health of your relationships and emotional life—and that's just for starters. Many women are surprised to learn that hormone health depends not on how old they are but on how healthy they are.

To give you the tools you need to master your hormones, I will revisit some lessons that you first learned in high school biology class.

Hormonal Facts and Figures

A hormone is a chemical messenger formed by an orchestra of highly talented players, such as the adrenal glands, the hypothalamus, the pituitary, the liver, the pancreas, the ovaries, and the thyroid. Hormones commute through your bloodstream via an information superhighway that connects the executive suites of your brain to the DNA managers working in your body's cells.

Hormones communicate with chemicals, called neurotransmitters, such as serotonin, dopamine, and norepinephrine, that are produced by our brains. These neurotransmitters greatly influence our energy levels, moods, and other bodily functions. Women's bodies contain female hormones such as estrogen, as well as male hormones such as testosterone and androstenodione, which are made by various endocrine glands and are responsible for libido, energy, and well-being.

Imagine your body as a city consisting of different commercial and residential neighborhoods, where several hundred trillion cells are busy living and working. Inside and outside the membranes of every cell, receptor sites function like elite clubs that can be entered only with special passwords. For any substance to enter the club and provide information to the DNA, the cells require the proper password. In this case, it is a hormone, which makes contact with a specific target cell and gains entry to the receptor site.

Once inside, the hormone delivers its biochemical messages for processing. For example, hormones have the power to switch various cellular functions on or off, such as telling the liver to make more blood glucose. They can orchestrate menstrual cycles and measure cellular activity throughout the body.

Depending on a woman's age, health, diet, fitness levels, and circumstances, her body will produce different hormones at different times of the day and the month. In most women, hormone levels peak in the early twenties and start descending after age twenty-five or so. Around age forty, hormone levels typically start to fluctuate, as the body moves beyond childbearing age and starts to prepare for life after menstruation, or postmenopause.

Because hormones affect the body in staggeringly complex ways, there are dozens of hormones that scientists have yet to fully understand. One of the most heavily researched female hormones, however, is estrogen, which is made in the ovaries and which circulates throughout the bloodstream. Besides activating a girl's metamorphosis into womanhood, estrogen creates the perfect conditions in the womb for the implantation and the nourishment of the early embryo. While estrogen acts as a growth hormone for breast, uterine, and ovarian tissue, it also fortifies the collagen layer of the skin, which improves elasticity and helps to prevent wrinkles. In addition, estrogen regulates mood and works many more health-enhancing wonders, which are detailed in chapter 2.

Women are often amazed when I tell them that the body produces more than two hundred different hormones every day. Just as certain nutrients from our food support specific aspects of mind/body health, each of your hundreds of hormones decisively influences specific body functions. In addition, hormone levels vary at different times of the day and night—they rise and fall throughout the twenty-four-hour cycle.

Your most famous hormones are undoubtedly the sex-related ones: estrogen, progesterone, and testosterone. Yes, even women produce the male hormone testosterone, and it's a lucky thing, too. Essential to healthy female sexual response and libido, testosterone also stokes energy and enhances general well-being. In most women, testosterone levels are doing fine until women reach a certain point in perimenopause, the six- to thirteen-year-long span that culminates in the last menstrual period.

Perimenopause may take place anywhere between the ages of forty and the late fifties, and symptoms vary from woman to woman. Irregular menstrual periods, missed periods, heavy or scanty bleeding, anxiety, and insomnia are some of the most common signs of perimenopause. Because these symptoms overlap with common PMS symptoms, the two conditions are often confused and thus misdiagnosed by health-care professionals. This book will help you pinpoint whether your mind/body conditions are caused by perimenopause or PMS. You will also find effective, safe, and evidence-based strategies for alleviating your symptoms.

You can develop a better sense of your exact condition(s) by completing the following questionnaires. Self-knowledge is empowering. Recording your symptoms is a great way to start balancing your hormones.

This first test increases your awareness about your current state of health. Please note that if you have had a hysterectomy, chances are high that you have a hormone imbalance.

If you check off three or more symptoms on the following Hormone Self-Assessment Test, you probably have unbalanced hormones. Please do not worry, as I will present solutions in the coming chapters that will help you take control of your health and eliminate any fears you may have now.

Hormone Self-Assessment Test

Check off any symptoms you are experiencing.

- ☐ have a history of antibiotic use
- ☐ frequently use prescription medications
- ☐ take synthetic hormones in a topical cream, a patch, or orally
- ☐ experience difficulty sleeping
- ☐ experience mood swings
- ☐ experience hot flashes
- ☐ experience low libido
- ☐ drink more than one glass of alcohol weekly
- ☐ drink caffeine daily
- ☐ experience exhaustion
- ☐ experience irregular menstrual cycles
- ☐ experience infertility
- ☐ experience frequent urination
- ☐ have vaginal dryness, pain
- ☐ experience painful intercourse
- ☐ have engorged breasts
- ☐ have milk production (not nursing)
- ☐ lack interest in sex
- ☐ have blurred vision
- ☐ experience headaches
- ☐ have acne and/or oily skin
- ☐ have aggressive feelings
- ☐ have overwhelming sexual urges
- ☐ have absence of menstrual flow for six or more months
- ☐ occasionally skip periods
- ☐ began menstruating after age sixteen
- ☐ have shrinking breasts
- ☐ have thinning pubic and armpit hair
- ☐ are unable to get pregnant
- ☐ had a miscarriage
- ☐ have excess facial hair
- ☐ have a poor sense of smell
- ☐ experience monthly abdominal pain without bleeding
- ☐ experience menstrual-type pain between menses
- ☐ have irregular time intervals between periods
- ☐ have menstrual cycles greater than thirty-two days
- ☐ have menstrual cycles less than twenty-four days
- ☐ have vaginal bleeding between periods
- ☐ experience progressively worse pain during periods
- ☐ have pain, cramps

The following Premenstrual Syndrome Self-Assessment Test will help you further define your physical and emotional health specifics so that you can better balance your hormones. Some of the following symptoms occur three days to two weeks prior to menstruation.

Premenstrual Syndrome Self-Assessment Test

Put a check mark beside everything that applies to you. Do you have . . . ?

☐ premenstrual tension

☐ painful menses (cramping, etc.)

☐ excessive or prolonged menstruation

☐ painful/tender breasts

☐ too frequent menstruation

☐ acne, worse at menses

☐ depressed feelings before menstruation

☐ vaginal discharge

☐ scanty or missed menses

☐ hysterectomy/ovaries removed

☐ depression

☐ insomnia

☐ abdominal bloating

☐ breast tenderness, swelling

☐ depression, irritability, nervousness

☐ feelings of being easy to anger, resentful

☐ a feeling of being easily over-whelmed

☐ nausea and/or vomiting

☐ diarrhea or constipation

☐ headache

☐ food cravings, binge eating

☐ back pain

☐ feelings of faintness

☐ clumsiness

☐ forgetfulness

☐ weight gain—water

☐ suicidal thoughts

Many women suffer from painful, tender swelling in the breasts and other disturbing symptoms that may be associated with fibrocystic breast disease. In my experience, this condition is widely under-diagnosed, yet easily treatable, so please take the following assessment to help you learn more about your body.

Dysplasia/Fibrocystic Syndrome Self-Assessment Test

Check off any symptoms you are experiencing.

- ☐ lumps that are painful, tender
- ☐ clear, gray, or yellow vaginal discharge
- ☐ vaginal bleeding after sex or between periods
- ☐ burning or itching on external genitalia
- ☐ urgent, painful urination
- ☐ lower abdominal or back pain
- ☐ heavy, watery, and bloody vaginal discharge
- ☐ heavy menstrual flow
- ☐ pelvic cramps

- ☐ thin, scant white vaginal discharge
- ☐ greenish yellow or offensive discharge
- ☐ cheesy white discharge
- ☐ breast lumps or swelling
- ☐ lumps that hurt just before period
- ☐ swelling under armpit
- ☐ change in breast size, shape
- ☐ white or slightly bloody vaginal discharge, one week prior to period
- ☐ current diagnosis of fibrocystic breast disease

Did you know that some women enter menopause in their late thirties, while others may keep menstruating regularly into their mid to late fifties? The following test will help you understand whether you have reached menopause.

Are You in Menopause?

Check off any symptoms that apply to you.

- ☐ irregular menstrual cycle
- ☐ excessive or prolonged menstruation
- ☐ too frequent menstruation
- ☐ acne, worse at menses
- ☐ scanty or missed menses
- ☐ hysterectomy/ovaries removed

- ☐ dry skin, hair, vagina
- ☐ lack of interest in sex
- ☐ mood swings, irritability
- ☐ depression, anxiety, nervousness
- ☐ craving for sweets, binge eating
- ☐ headaches or dizziness

- [ ] painful intercourse
- [ ] sudden hot flashes
- [ ] spontaneous sweating
- [ ] shortness of breath and/or heart palpitations
- [ ] unpredictable vaginal bleeding
- [ ] difficulty holding urine
- [ ] difficulty sleeping
- [ ] mental fogginess
- [ ] vaginal pain and/or itching
- [ ] thin, scant white vaginal discharge

- [ ] low back and/or hip pain
- [ ] breast tenderness, pain, or tingling, prickling sensation
- [ ] easy bruising, loss of skin tone
- [ ] thinning armpit and pubic hair
- [ ] stopped menstruating
- [ ] breasts beginning to shrink, sag
- [ ] abnormal growth of hair above lip

Because critical hormones like testosterone are made in the ovaries, it's vital to check out your ovarian function. Here's an ovarian dysfunction self-assessment test to guide and educate you about your body. Just check off your symptoms and any diagnosis you have had.

Ovarian Dysfunction Self-Assessment

Check off all that apply to you. Do you have . . . ?

- [ ] vaginal dryness, pain
- [ ] painful intercourse
- [ ] engorged breasts
- [ ] milk production (not nursing)
- [ ] lack of interest in sex
- [ ] blurred vision
- [ ] headache
- [ ] acne and/or oily skin
- [ ] aggressive feelings
- [ ] overwhelming sexual urges
- [ ] absence of menstrual flow for six or more months

- [ ] occasional missed periods
- [ ] menstruation that began after age sixteen
- [ ] shrinking breasts
- [ ] thinning pubic and armpit hair
- [ ] inability to get pregnant
- [ ] miscarriage
- [ ] excess facial hair
- [ ] poor sense of smell
- [ ] monthly abdominal pain without bleeding

☐ menstrual-type pain between menses

☐ irregular time intervals between periods

☐ menstrual cycles greater than thirty-two days

☐ menstrual cycles less than twenty-four days

☐ vaginal bleeding between periods

☐ pain during periods that is getting progressively worse

☐ pain, cramps

As you read this book and follow its detoxification and hormone-balancing strategies, your symptoms should improve. Refer back to these quizzes to check your original answers, which will help clarify any improvement in endocrine functioning and hormone health.

If you find that you're experiencing a hormone imbalance, then you're not alone. Today, about 40 million women in the United States are either in perimenopause or are postmenopausal. In the United States, the average age of menopause is currently about fifty-two, with a range from forty-five to the late fifties. I have seen women who experienced menopause in their late thirties, either naturally or as a result of surgical hysterectomy. Over the last four decades or so, the medical profession and the pharmaceutical industry have treated per-imenopausal and postmenopausal symptoms (caused by hormone imbalances) as diseases that require synthetic hormone replacement therapy (HRT) drugs.

I have been a health provider for almost twenty-five years and have never recommended a drug. Nor do I find them able to cure any degenerative disease. I believe that a combination of homeopathic remedies, careful diet, exercise, meditation, and naturally derived nutritional substances are the best choice for PMS, perimenopausal, or postmenopausal symptoms.

I see perimenopause and the stages beyond as highlights of the female journey and growth process. I say *growth* process, rather than aging process, because not only are women living longer than ever before, they are living smarter. Recent medical advances and more healthful lifestyles mean that women enjoy a better quality of life—as well as greater longevity—than their mothers or grandmothers did.

The Scientific Evidence against Conventional HRT

In the United States most women with a uterus who report symptoms such as Sarah's are put on conventional HRT, which combines synthetic estrogen with progestin, also known as synthetic progesterone. An estimated 13.5 to 16 million women in the United States use HRT, synthetic estrogen either alone or combined with synthetic progesterone.

The most commonly prescribed synthetic estrogen is called Premarin, a collection of over twenty different conjugated equine estrogens made from the urine of pregnant horses. Premarin, the oldest synthetic estrogen, has been on the market since 1944. The name Premarin is an acronym derived from a weirdly unforgettable product, pregnant mare's urine. Whoa! Logic dictates that it is wholly unnatural for women to consume hormones sourced from the urine of pregnant mares. If you drop a little water on a Premarin tablet, the pungent aroma of horse pee will help you smell my point.

Nevertheless, women have willingly swallowed this stuff for decades under the direction of their physicians. Premarin is one of the world's most widely prescribed drugs and is sold alone or combined with another hormone in the drugs Prempro and Premphase.

Progestin, usually Provera (medroxyprogesterone acetate), is combined with estrogen because it prevents Premarin from causing excessive tissue growth inside the uterus, which over time can lead to cancer of the endometrium, or uterine lining. Produced in the laboratory, Provera is markedly different from naturally occurring progesterone. The combination of Premarin and Provera is called Prempro. Synthetic hormones like Prempro place a tremendous stress on your liver and the other players in your body's detoxification system.

Conventional HRT's health risks made front-page news back in July 2002, when the largest and longest U.S. study of HRT ever conducted came to a dramatically premature end. The study was halted three years ahead of schedule because participants (16,608 healthy women, ages fifty to seventy-nine years) taking synthetic estrogen and progestin were found to be at significantly higher risk for breast cancer, heart attack, stroke, and blood clots than were women in the placebo group.

This historic study was sponsored by the Women's Health Initiative (WHI), funded by the National Heart, Lung, and Blood Institute of the National Institutes of Health (NIH). Results published in the *Journal of the American Medical Association* specified that women who take estrogen and progestin for more than five years expose themselves to the risk of a

- 26 percent increase in breast cancer
- 22 percent increase in cardiovascular disease
- 41 percent increase in strokes
- 100 percent increase in blood clots

In its press release on the cancellation of the trial, the NIH sounded an exceptionally clear warning regarding the dangers of taking estrogen plus progestin. The study results offered irrefutable proof that "on balance the harm was greater than the benefits." Contradicting popular medical belief, the study also reported that HRT's effects on osteoporosis and dementia prevention appeared negligible. WHI researchers, who rarely recommend any actions except more studies, secured their place in the annals of medical history by advising doctors to be very cautious about prescribing HRT to their patients. This unprecedented action confirmed that the American public should avoid taking HRT because of its many dangerous side effects.

Physicians and health researchers also have compelling reasons to wonder whether the widespread practice of prescribing Prempro over the last three decades is linked to the rise in U.S. breast cancer rates. According to the National Alliance of Breast Cancer Organizations (NABCO), "based on the current life expectancy for women in the United States, one out of nine women will develop breast cancer in her lifetime—a risk that was one out of 14 in 1960." That clearly adds up to a dangerous increase.

The WHI results came as a shocking wake-up call to the approximately 6 million U.S. women who were taking estrogen plus progestin in 2002. Understandably, the results also alarmed women who had used it in the past. It is only natural that they felt (or continue to feel) angered and frightened by the findings. When the study's disease risk numbers were evaluated with respect to the 6 million women in the United States who were currently taking HRT, it meant that tens of thousands of women were at increased risk of serious illness or disease. The truth contained in these figures is unassailable: taking HRT may seriously endanger your health.

Following the publication of the WHI results in July 2002, hormone therapy prescriptions declined in successive months. Relative to January–June 2002, prescriptions from January to June 2003 declined by 66 percent for Prempro and 33 percent for Premarin.

Along with alerting women to the potential dangers of conventional HRT, the WHI scandal woke up millions to the fact that even though a drug is FDA-approved, it may never have been thoroughly researched in large-scale, double-blind, placebo-controlled trials. In other words, a drug's relative safety may be in question long after it is FDA-approved, and like HRT, the drug may even negatively affect your health.

That HRT was FDA-approved before being adequately researched is undeniable and a major reason why women were encouraged to take HRT for so long. So is the fact that over the years, numerous small studies have shown that long-term, constant HRT helps to preserve bone mass, an important concern among women over fifty. You can't blame physicians or patients for wanting to prevent osteoporosis with a drug that has been found to help prevent it. But then again, more recent research about HRT's effects may not have reached all of the doctors who treat postmenopausal women, or the women themselves.

Although the osteoporosis connection is one of the murkiest reasons why women have gladly taken conventional and other forms of HRT (and continue to take them, despite an awareness of the risks), the marketing machine behind these drugs cannot be discounted. Over the last few decades, pharmaceutical companies have led physicians and women to believe that Prempro and other forms of HRT can help a woman feel and look younger, sexier, and more vibrant. Some pharmaceutical firms and physicians have also promoted its potential for preventing heart disease.

Recently, however, the Heart and Estrogen/Progestin Replacement Study (HERS) study and the Estrogen Replacement in Atherosclerosis (ERA) trial found that HRT, instead of reducing the risk of heart disease for midlife women, actually increases the risk.

Larger research trials sounded even more alarms about the mortal dangers of taking Prempro. In the United Kingdom, a study of more than a million women who took Prempro found that it could double a woman's risk of developing breast cancer and increase the risk of dying from breast cancer by 22 percent.

This study found that for every thousand women who use HRT for ten years beginning at age fifty, there will be an additional nineteen cases of cancer in those using Prempro and an extra five in women using estrogen-only HRT. The researchers estimated that twenty thousand cases of breast cancer have occurred in the United Kingdom over the last decade in women from ages fifty to sixty-four because of HRT. It was estimated that fifteen thousand were caused by Prempro. Statistics on HRT-caused breast cancer, stroke, uterine cancer, or heart disease in American women have yet to be compiled. Given that the U.S. population is roughly six times that of the United Kingdom, could it be possible that 120,000 cases of breast cancer in the United States have been caused by HRT in the last decade?

Toxic Effects of Some Hormones Used in Conventional HRT

Even for women who can tolerate HRT without experiencing any disturbing side effects (and most cannot), it's worth noting that HRT never addresses the real cause of their hormone imbalance. I've worked with thousands of patients and reviewed their hormone saliva tests for their health providers; this has shown me that many women who use conventional HRT develop toxically high levels of progesterone and/or estrogen, DHEA, and so on.

As a result, they report many uncomfortable symptoms that clear up once they stop using HRT and stay on my program for at least three months. Toxically high levels of progesterone, estrogen, and other hormones are so prevalent among women on HRT that clinical laboratories that analyze saliva tests print them out on every lab report as a standard entry. Progesterone toxicity is known to cause weight gain, hair loss, loss of libido, depression, excessive hot flashes, and hormone system dysfunction.

Likewise, estrogen toxicity is known to trigger such dangerous conditions as breast lumps/uterus problems, ovarian problems (such as tumors, fibroids, and so on), cancer, heart disease, blood clots, weight gain, excessive facial hair, and gallstones.

In various studies, 20 percent of women who take estrogen and testosterone HRT have been found to develop mild hair growth (the medical term is *hirsutism*). Although hirsutism is dose-dependent and reversible, developing facial hair at any age is a negative. Since women tend to grow more facial and chin hair with age, it can be quite depressing if facial hair sprouts during perimenopause or later. Testosterone in high doses has also been found to deepen women's voices.

Now that you have read the sobering news about HRT, you may wonder whether so-called natural hormones are safer for your body or perhaps more effective.

The Truth about "Natural" and "Bio-Identical" Hormones

The fact that authoritative studies have proved that conventional HRT drugs are dangerous or ineffective is often used to justify taking so-called natural, bio-identical hormones. With all the fear and confusion surrounding the dangers of HRT, the idea of taking "natural" or "bio-identical" hormones may sound very comforting to you. I know that the thought of taking "natural" estrogen, progesterone, and testosterone has soothed the fears of many of my patients.

The only problem is, these women ended up in my office because the so-called natural hormones that they took were ineffective or caused unpleasant side effects such as weight gain, brain fog, insomnia, heart palpitations, and so on. Although many famous physicians and celebrities may endorse "natural" hormones, they consistently gloss over the fact that "natural" or "bio-identical" hormones are synthesized in a laboratory. These synthetic hormones are just as foreign to your system as are prescription drug–based hormone replacement therapy (HRT) formulas.

Moreover, people who endorse "natural" hormones also fail to address the reality that women who take these "natural" substances (even wild yam progesterone cream) routinely develop toxically high hormone levels, which can potentially be problematic. As toxically high hormone levels factor into the many thousands of cancers that are linked to synthetic HRT use, it seems likely that toxic levels of hormones resulting from "natural" hormone use may also create potentially dangerous consequences.

Medically Proven Dangers of Using "Natural" Hormone Creams

One of the first studies on how "natural" hormone creams affect hormone levels was conducted by Dr. Anne Hermann at Bassett Healthcare in Cooperstown, New York. Presenting the results at the March 2004 conference of the American Society for Clinical Pharmacology and Therapeutics in Florida, Dr. Hermann reported that women who used Pro-Gest "natural" progesterone cream to relieve hot flashes and night sweats later had the same high levels of progesterone in their bloodstreams as a group that took the hormone pill Prometrium.

"Millions of women are using these creams, thinking that because they're natural and sold over the counter, they are safe," Dr. Hermann told the *New York Times*. "The reality is that they are putting themselves at risk." According to a Food and Drug Administration spokeswoman, Susan Cruzan, also quoted in the same article, "Until research shows otherwise," "natural" progesterone is considered to involve similar health risks as its synthetic version.

Here's another red flag: on the thousands of saliva test reports that I've analyzed and collected, the hormonal reference ranges for women who use wild yam (progesterone) liposome creams are extraordinarily high. Thus, although doctors know how common it is for women who use "natural" creams to have off-the-chart progesterone levels, they continue to prescribe these products anyway.

It's essential for you to realize that progesterone cream, whether "bio-identical" or not, may cause a woman's body to harbor more than fifty times the normal amount of progesterone. This situation could lead to serious health and/or quality of life consequences, such as dramatically worse perimenopausal or menopausal symptoms or the development of breast cancers or other diseases. But before we go any further, we need to take a good look at what "natural" or "bio-identical" hormones are made of, so that you can see for yourself how healthful an alternative they actually are.

As I mentioned earlier, all of the "natural" or "bio-identical" hormones prescribed today are synthesized in a laboratory from soybeans or wild yams, two substances that are about as native to your body as the urine of pregnant mares or Provera is. Whether they come in the form of capsules, gels, sublingual drops, suppositories, or topical and vaginal gels and creams, "natural" hormones are processed chemically and made into hormones that are supposedly identical to those produced by your body.

You may wonder how these so-called natural substances can be identical to your hormones if they are manufactured in a laboratory. The truth is, they cannot. It follows that in this case, the term *natural hormones* is a misnomer.

When a woman starts taking "bio-identical" hormones, her health-care provider may need to change the formula several times before finding one that relieves her symptoms. This process can be frustrating, tiring, and expensive, as it may require multiple visits to the health-care provider, along with added charges for hormone blood or saliva tests, to find a formula that balances the individual's hormones.

It must also be noted here that when hormonal levels seesaw, this strains the adrenal glands and causes them to secrete abnormal amounts of the stress hormone cortisol (you will read much more about cortisol in the coming chapters). When cortisol levels are abnormal, this burdens the entire endocrine system and makes achieving hormonal balance all the more challenging.

Another "natural" hormone fact to remember: because hormone levels change in response to stressful events, diet, and lifestyle habits, a formula may work for just a few months and then lose its efficacy. This is because the hormonal profile that the formula was designed to address may have reconfigured into an entirely new shape. With the old formula obsolete, you're back at square one, seeking relief for mind/body symptoms.

In the case of "natural" hormones, physicians have defined the word *natural* to suit their agenda—an agenda that requires patients to keep coming into the office for regular appointments. Your body has no such agenda. It feels and knows the difference between its own hormones and supplemental ones, just as it can identify transplanted organs and tell the difference between natural sunlight and artificial light.

Although many physicians and health-care professionals tout the benefits of "natural" hormones, even less research data exists for them than for conventional HRT! To add insult to injury, there is also a complete lack of data showing how (or whether) "natural hormones" may help prevent breast or other reproductive cancers or may provide therapeutic approaches to these diseases.

The "natural" hormone research void is mainly due to the fact that these types of hormones are not patented substances. They are not made by large pharmaceutical companies, which can easily afford to invest millions in scientific trials to obtain medical-use approval for the patented drugs that they own. And since no one company owns a specific "natural" hormone—as, say, Wyeth-Ayerst owns Premarin—there is a lack of incentive for "natural" hormone manufacturers to bankroll placebo-controlled, double-blind studies, which are costly, labor-intensive, and time-consuming.

Another important point is that although "natural" hormones are legal, the FDA does not approve them. Please remember for your own sake, and for the sake of all women who take them, that any claims made about them by health-care professionals, health food store clerks, or others have never been confirmed by research.

Because so-called natural hormones are believed to be identical to the hormones your body produces, because they are prescribed by physicians in customized dosages, and because they are prepared by compounding pharmacies with individual care, "natural" hormones are touted by many physicians as being safer and far superior to conventional HRT drugs. Nevertheless, as of this writing, no scientist knows whether taking natural estrogen with progesterone is more or less risky than taking conventional HRT.

If you're wondering whether long-term natural hormone use carries increased cancer risks, no one knows that, either. The same goes for over-the-counter (OTC) hormones sold in health food stores, such as DHEA (dehydroepiandrosterone). DHEA is essential for optimal brain and endocrine system functioning; it is also crucial for maintaining immunity and energy. Because it can be converted into various steroid hormones, including estrogen and testosterone, DHEA is called a precursor hormone.

In the body, DHEA is made by the adrenal glands. As DHEA sulfate, it travels to various tissues, including the breasts, the endometrium (uterine lining), and the muscles. Upon arrival in the tissues, it's converted to the appropriate sex hormone for that area. Ingesting DHEA can cause the body to lose its capacity to make its own DHEA, just as taking any other hormone supplement can shut down production of a specific hormone. And, as with using any form of HRT, DHEA supplementation can allow toxically high levels of the hormone to accumulate, potentially triggering various health problems.

In addition to accelerating the growth of existing tumors, scientists have observed that DHEA can cause facial hair growth and a deepening of the voice in women. I tell all of my patients to have a saliva test to check DHEA (or any other hormone) levels before they take supplemental hormones. You can obtain this test from a holistic health-care provider. (See the Resource Guide.)

On the plus side (and it's a potentially huge plus), a clinical study of female patients with the painful autoimmune disease lupus, conducted at Stanford University, found that 200 mg of DHEA a day markedly relieved symptoms, while women on placebo reported no improvement. If you've been diagnosed with lupus, you may want to discuss DHEA supplementation with your health-care provider.

Like DHEA, pregnenolone is another precursor hormone that cannot be patented. In the body, it's synthesized directly from cholesterol. The brain and the peripheral nerves manufacture huge amounts of it. Because it's made in the brain, pregnenolone is often referred to as a neurohormone.

The pregnenolone that you buy over the counter is synthesized from yams in the laboratory and sold in health food stores and on the Internet. Pregnenolone is the mother of all steroidal hormones (also known as sex hormones); even DHEA is made from it. Scientists are still unsure about how pregnenolone affects the full spectrum of human health. While there are some medical or psychiatric conditions where it can be used temporarily and then stopped, nothing is known about how it may affect PMS, depression, and other common medical conditions.

Although I know many physicians who prescribe pregnenolone for hormone replacement therapy, please note that no studies have ever evaluated whether it's an appropriate treatment. Therefore, scientists know nothing about how long-term use of pregnenolone as hormone replacement therapy may affect the body. Even physicians who specialize in hormone balancing have noted in print that most of the pregnenolone dosages available in over-the-counter products are too high for regular daily consumption and can lead to toxic side effects.

Pregnenolone's side effects may include heart palpitations, over-stimulation and insomnia, heart rhythm irregularities, irritability, anger, anxiety, acne, headaches, scalp hair loss, and thyroid gland disturbances.

You Can Save Yourself from the Dangers of HRT

I hope that you now have a healthy appreciation of the potential dangers of both conventional and so-called natural HRT.

In the following chapters, I'll take you step-by-step through my program and teach you how to achieve hormone balance without incurring the side effects and the potentially dangerous health risks associated with all forms of HRT.

Step 1 Action Plan

1. Eliminate all fear through education and knowledge. Learn about your body and health choices. Take notes and take responsibility for empowering and healing yourself.
2. Keep reading this book and complete the self-assessment tests in each chapter.
3. Follow the action plans at the end of each chapter.
4. Study the homeopathic chart in chapter 7 and take action to eliminate your symptoms.
5. Follow the detoxification guidelines in chapter 3 and the Endocrine-Rebuilding Diet.
6. Use the Nutrient List according to your symptoms.
7. Take a Five Element Saliva Test. (This tests hormones according to the Chinese Body Clock, which you'll learn more about later in the book; also see the Resource Guide.)

Step 2

Understanding Your Hormones and Why They Go Out of Balance

Christine, age forty-one, was a successful attorney who had endured heavy PMS her entire adult life. Like many professional women I work with, she rarely prepared her own meals, ate healthful snacks, drank enough water, or exercised regularly. Christine existed mainly on fast, processed foods and lots of coffee—the Standard American Diet, which health-care professionals fittingly refer to as SAD. Although she had a strong and generous spirit, Christine felt, by her own admission, "fried," and her PMS was getting unbearable.

I strongly suspected that her symptoms were lifestyle related. After years of Christine's working overtime, exercising too little, and consuming mass quantities of sugar, caffeine, refined carbohydrates, and chemical-laden foods, her endocrine system lacked the energy, the nutrients, the rest, and the exercise it needed to function properly.

Hormone saliva tests confirmed that all six of her adrenal cortisol levels, including her liver testing time, were low, indicating that her sex hormones were depleted and unbalanced. Obviously, her long-term sugar and caffeine habits contributed strongly to her condition. (Sugar and refined carbohydrate intake had made her blood sugar levels soar and then plummet for years. It has been proved in various studies that caffeine negatively affects adrenal gland function and cortisol levels.)

Christine's ob/gyn suggested that she take birth control pills, but she had already tried these briefly several years ago under another doctor's direction, and they failed to remedy her PMS. Now, Christine understood that taking birth control pills might expose her to health risks she would rather avoid. Much to Christine's relief, I explained that she didn't have to take pills to get her hormones back in balance. Instead, like many of my patients before her, she could markedly improve her mind/body health by cutting out caffeine, sugar, excessive carbohydrates, and chemically processed foods. Christine followed my directions precisely (if only every patient were as cooperative as she) and called after just three weeks to report that she felt dramatically better.

In addition to following a homeopathic revitalization program and using my recipes, which contain whole, fresh, nutritious organic foods, Christine practiced stress-management techniques to help reduce her PMS symptoms and improve her mental and physical energy. She also maintained a regular exercise regimen for the first time in her life and found that it made her feel calmer and more rested.

After just two months, Christine ecstatically announced that her PMS symptoms had decreased dramatically. She was sleeping better than she had in years and even lost a few pounds without counting calories. "My mood swings are gone and I feel I can handle challenges better," she told me. "I feel like I've been tuned up." That's exactly what my program did for her mentally, emotionally, and physically.

Your hormones are like an orchestra: if one instrument is out of tune, the whole production struggles to maintain harmony. Finding the source of the discord takes patience and skill, but in this book, you'll learn how to be your own hormone detective. As the first action step, we'll work on strengthening and balancing your endocrine system, which produces two hundred hormones and is exquisitely sensitive.

Each hormone greatly influences how well the other hormones work. Just as there are many reasons why an orchestra can fall out of tune, there are numerous reasons why your hormones may become either deficient or excessively high. (You may have heard of estrogen dominance. Overly high estrogen levels are common among perimenopausal women.) Before I help you discover any potential hormone imbalances and possible causes, we're going to tour the endocrine system. Once you learn how its glands and hormones team up to help you stay healthy, sexy, and strong, you'll understand how profoundly endocrine function affects your PMS, your periods, and your overall health.

In this chapter, you'll take self-assessment tests that will yield important clues about your hormone health. You'll gain valuable information on common hormone-related conditions that can affect reproductive health, such as endometriosis, which afflicts at least 10 percent of all U.S. women and millions more worldwide. Most important, by the time you finish this chapter, you'll understand the health habits and the circumstances that can cause endocrine breakdown, and you'll learn how to stop it.

Endocrine System 101

Think of the endocrine system as one of your body's main power grids. It's responsible for many crucial bodily processes and consists of various organs and glands that secrete hormones. The endocrine system works by releasing hormones that, in turn, trigger actions in specific target cells. For any cell to respond to a particular hormone, it must already possess a specific receptor that recognizes this hormone. Receptors are proteins made by cells that allow the cells to identify substances, such as hormones, in their environment. Each hormone simply binds to its receptor, and this activates the cell.

Hormone levels vary at different times of the day and are influenced by factors such as diet, stress, exercise, infection, and lack of sleep. Changes in the balance of fluid and minerals in blood also influence hormone levels.

Endocrine Glands and Hormone Production

Like a fine gold chain woven of many delicate links, the function of each endocrine gland greatly affects the overall strength and resilience of the endocrine system. To begin our tour, we'll start with the pituitary gland.

The pituitary activates multiple glands and secretes several hormones. The pituitary is the size of a pea and is located beneath the hypothalamus in a small, bony cavity at the base of the brain. I call it the hormonal diva because it rules your endocrine system with high energy and star power.

Did you know that this hormonal diva generates ten essential hormones that keep you feeling energetic and sexy? They are:

Oxytocin: Promotes uterine contraction and milk ejection in nursing women; responds to the sucking reflex and estradiol.

Vasopressin (antidiuretic hormone or ADH): Regulates blood pressure and increases the body's fluid balance.

Melanocyte-stimulating hormone (MSH): Controls skin pigmentation.

Corticotropin: Also referred to as adrenocorticotropin or ACTH; stimulates cells of the adrenal glands to increase steroid synthesis and secretion.

Lipotropin: Also known as LPH; increases the fatty acid release from fat cells.

Thyrotropin (thyroid-stimulating hormone or TSH): Activates thyroid follicle cells to stimulate thyroid hormone synthesis.

Growth hormone: Often called human growth hormone or hGH. This increases the release of insulin-like growth factor-1 (IGF-1), along with cell growth and bone health. It's also a general anabolic stimulant. By age sixty, most people will have approximately 80 percent less growth hormone in their system than when they were twenty. Signs of hGH reduction include increased body fat, increased anxiety, social isolation, poor general health, and lack of positive well-being.

I'd like to clarify a few facts about hGH supplementation, because it's such a controversial and trendy subject. Baby boomers seeking to maintain their youthful edge are taking hGH for its many rejuvenating and antiaging effects. Physicians who are antiaging specialists prescribe hGH; it typically costs up to $170 per day.

Here's what you need to know about hGH. To begin with, hGH can help to improve brain activity and function. It can promote weight loss, while producing more muscle cells and maximizing muscle growth. Naturally occurring hGH supports immune system and thymus gland performance, while also strengthening connective tissue and reducing injury risk. Along with elevating energy and mood, hGH improves lung function, which raises oxygen levels in the bloodstream. In my opinion, however, the health risks never justify taking supplemental hGH, for this is still hormone replacement.

Toxic levels of hGH can trigger swelling of the soft tissues in the body; abnormal growth of the hands, the feet, and the facial features; high blood pressure and increased perspiration; plus excessive hair growth. In addition, hGH may feed tumor growth in the body. Therefore, it's extremely important that a physician supervise you while you take it. Homeopathic hGH would be a wiser choice, or specific amino acid formulas.

Prolactin (PRL): Stimulates mammary gland function and milk synthesis; increases ovarian progesterone synthesis.

Luteinizing hormone (LH): Induces ovulation and activates progesterone secretion to support egg implantation and pregnancy.

Follicle-stimulating hormone (FSH): Promotes ovarian follicle development and ovulation; increases estrogen production.

The pituitary is made up of two lobes: the anterior and the posterior. The anterior pituitary regulates protein synthesis, tissue growth, and immune stimulation. It affects hormone demand and utilization, as well as protein and fat metabolism.

The posterior pituitary works in concert with the adrenals, much like an orchestra's drum and bass. This part of the pituitary secretes oxytocin, which stimulates the uterine contractions of labor, as well as milk secretion for nursing a baby. The posterior pituitary also secretes ADH, which regulates water balance and causes sodium retention via the kidneys.

Circumstances that can cause the pituitary to operate at less-than-optimal levels may include prolonged periods of emotional stress; head injury; heavy metal toxicity, including mercury toxicity from dental amalgam fillings; nuclear radiation; legal and illegal drug abuse; neurotransmitter imbalance; and pesticide and insecticide exposure.

An executive partner to the pituitary is the hypothalamus, connected to the pituitary by a slender thread of nerve tissue. The hypothalamus exerts powerful effects on the human body. Regulating body temperature and the autonomic nervous system (you'll learn more about this later in the chapter), the hypothalamus plays a leading role in processing emotions. For these and other reasons, the hypothalamus is called the "director" gland of the brain.

The hypothalamus has a heavy hormone connection: seven hypothalamic hormones are released into the system that connects the hypothalamus and the pituitary, which in turn activate pituitary sites to release eight hormones.

Here's the skinny on hypothalamic hormones:

Corticotropin-releasing factor (also known as CRF or CRH): Activates corticotropin and lipoprotein release.

Gonadotropin-releasing factor (commonly abbreviated as GnRF or GnRH): Stimulates the release of luteinizing hormone and follicle-stimulating hormone. (These two hormones are necessary for conception.)

Prolactin-releasing factor (PRF): Stimulates prolactin release.

Prolactin-release inhibiting factor (PRIF): Inhibits prolactin release.

Growth hormone–releasing factor (GRF or GRH): Stimulates growth hormone secretion.

Somatostatin (SIF): Also referred to as growth hormone–release inhibiting factor or GIF; inhibits GH and TSH secretion.

Thyrotropin-releasing factor (TRF or TRH): Stimulates secretion of thyroid-stimulating hormone and prolactin secretion.

As with the pituitary, many conditions may interfere with normal hypothalamus function. These include prolonged periods of emotional stress, neurotransmitter imbalance, exposure to mercury and pesticides, legal and illegal drug abuse, head injury, and nuclear radiation, which also toxifies the body.

Located between the eyes and deep within the brain is the pineal gland. It's behind that area on the forehead that many yogic traditions call the third eye. The pineal is a tiny gland that registers light and tells the brain and the optic nerve how light or dark the environment is. The pineal secretes melatonin, a hormone involved in helping you feel calm and stay asleep. The pineal also communicates with the ovaries. Studies have shown that low melatonin levels can be brought back in balance by our sleeping in a pitch-black room every night for six weeks or more. (This should be continued to maintain melatonin levels.)

The Thyroid Gland

The butterfly-shaped thyroid gland is a major player in the endocrine system. It sits at the base of the neck and generates hormones that are essential for growth and health throughout all stages of life. In broad strokes, here are your thyroid hormones and their job descriptions:

Thyroglobulin: A storage form of thyroid hormone. TSH from the pituitary causes the conversion of thyroglobulin into the thyroid hormones T4 and T3, which are necessary for normal growth and development, for sexual maturation, and for the regulation of metabolism.

Thyroxine and triiodothyronine: Regulate body temperature and metabolism; respond to TSH and stimulate oxidation in many cells.

Calcitonin: Regulates blood calcium and protein metabolism.

Calcitonin gene-related peptide: Dilates blood vessels.

Parathyroid hormone (PTH): Regulates calcium and protein metabolism; promotes bone health.

Nearly all body cells are targets of thyroid hormones, which indicates how essential they are to our well-being. The thyroid also promotes digestion and the secretion of digestive juices. In addition to increasing the body's metabolic activity rate, the thyroid stimulates protein synthesis, growth, and development and secretes calcitonin, which lowers blood calcium.

The thyroid is often a cause of hormone imbalance, and thyroid disease is extremely common. In fact, a study evaluating the prevalence of thyroid disease indicated that more than 13 million Americans may be unaware that they have a thyroid condition, even though the disease is undermining their short- and long-term health. (That's about 5 percent of the population.)

When the thyroid gland malfunctions, it can become underactive (hypothyroidism) or overactive (hyperthyroidism). Either condition leads to many of the symptoms that women associate with dysfunctional sex hormones. (In traditional Chinese medical theory, the thyroid and the adrenal glands are on the same energetic axis. For this reason, it's important that they be treated simultaneously to help promote hormone balance. I use homeopathic combinations for this.)

Like many women, you may suspect that you have a thyroid problem. You may also have heard reports on how inaccurate thyroid blood testing can be. In fact, new research strongly suggests that saliva testing can produce a more accurate measurement of thyroid-stimulating hormone. A saliva test measures the hormones that are unbound or freely circulating throughout your body.

Some doctors choose to use hormone urine tests. A major drawback of this method is that a urine test reports what you lose and excrete every day, rather than the hormone levels that actually circulate through your body. Hormone urine tests may be strongly influenced by caffeine intake, stress levels, diet, and other factors that affect hormone levels. Moreover, the hormone urine test does not measure at the two-hour intervals of the Chinese Five Element Body Clock method. (You'll find more on this later in the book.)

Please complete the Thyroid Self-Assessment Test on page 36 to help determine whether you may have a hypo- or hyperfunctioning thyroid. If you check only one symptom in each list, your thyroid may be working just fine. If you check a few symptoms, your thyroid function could be off-kilter. Thyroid symptoms are quite common and are often misread as signs of perimenopause, aging, depression, or stress. What's more, even when women do seek medical help for hypothyroidism, they often don't undergo the nuanced testing that's required for an accurate diagnosis. Take the case of my patient Katrina, who e-mailed me the following:

My doctor is using my basal body temperature (BBT) as a guide to determine whether I've met my optimum thyroid medication level. I take my temperature under my arm first thing upon waking for three days in a row and write it down. I recently read that this is much more accurate than the blood tests (target range between 97.8 to 98.2), so why don't other doctors use this method? I had never heard of using the BBT until I went to this doctor.

My BBT for the three days ranged from 95.6 to 96.8, though my TSH level at my last doctor was in the normal range. (I have since fired that doctor.) After that TSH test, my new doctor increased my thyroid meds, and my BBT is still low.

What is really going on? Please let me know your opinion about the BBT testing method and whether saliva testing would be more accurate.

Katrina's story highlights how difficult it can be to help people with underactive thyroids. As I told her, there is considerable evidence that current blood tests lack sensitivity and accuracy, whether they're being used to diagnose hypothyroidism or to manage and monitor a case under treatment. To ensure that I make safe and effective recommendations in my private practice and in second-opinion sessions with patients of other practitioners, I insist that basal body temperature (BBT) and TSH saliva tests form part of the equation.

If you're wondering whether your health problems are due totally or in part to an underactive thyroid, BBT and TSH salivary tests are necessary, along with a full inventory of symptoms, family history, related conditions, and physical signs of abnormality.

If you've been diagnosed with hypothyroidism, the BBT test is an additional confirmation that helps to determine whether you are reacting positively to the homeopathic remedies, the improved nutrition, and the right dosage. Be aware that Katrina's assertion that the BBT test is "much more accurate than the blood tests" is simply not true for all patients.

Therefore, you must piece together many clues to complete the puzzle and determine whether to treat a health problem as a low thyroid issue or, if you're presently under medical care, whether to add or change medication or supplements. If your doctor says that your TSH blood test is normal, and you really feel unwell, you should check your BBT and get a TSH salivary test. For more information on accurately diagnosing your thyroid problems, see the detailed instructions in appendix A.

Thyroid Self-Assessment Test

Please take time to consider which of the symptoms listed in the following two sections apply to you. If you check more than four symptoms in either section, this may indicate that you are possibly hypothyroid or hyperthyroid. In that event, I suggest you do a Barnes underarm test, as detailed in appendix A.

Check off the hypothyroid symptoms that apply to you.

☐ puffy face and swollen eyelids   ☐ cold hands and feet
☐ dry skin and hair   ☐ tendency to gain weight and
☐ hair loss   obesity

☐ irregular menstrual periods
☐ morning stiffness
☐ constipation
☐ muscle and joint pain
☐ fatigue
☐ depression
☐ headaches or migraine (check for corn allergy)
☐ neurotic behavior
☐ sensitivity to cold

☐ slowness
☐ sleepiness
☐ low energy
☐ frequent infections
☐ circulatory problems
☐ poor memory and/or concentration
☐ chronic skin problems
☐ eczema
☐ psoriasis

If you have a few symptoms on the previous checklist, I recommend a combination homeopathic adrenal/thyroid formula that can balance the thyroid and the adrenals. You'll find these in the homeopathic chart in chapter 7. In addition, seaweeds such as kelp, kombu, dulse, hijiki, and wakame have been proven to raise the metabolism of hypothyroid individuals.

Check off the hyperthyroid symptoms that apply to you.

☐ thin face
☐ oily skin and hair
☐ hair loss
☐ warm hands and feet
☐ trembling fingers
☐ tachycardia (excessively rapid heartbeat)
☐ weight loss with muscle weakness
☐ fatigue with muscle weakness

☐ sleep disorders
☐ insomnia
☐ nervousness
☐ anxiety
☐ overheating
☐ sweating
☐ diarrhea
☐ quick heart palpitations
☐ menstrual disorders

If you have several symptoms on the previous checklist, I recommend the following: eliminate all stimulants, such as caffeine, chocolate, sugar, and seaweed, because these can exacerbate the condition. Take 50 mg once or twice a day of vitamin B-complex, from whole food sources, as this calms the body. In addition, refer to the homeopathic chart in chapter 7 for remedies that may help to balance your symptoms.

The Adrenal Glands

The next stop on our endocrine odyssey is the adrenal glands. These make your heart race when you're excited, stressed, scared, or in love. The adrenals release many hormones, including adrenaline, which makes you feel buzzed and jumpy when you consume too much caffeine. The adrenal glands are instrumental in making you feel exhausted, burned out, or fried, and they also help to power hot flashes and other vexing menopausal symptoms. Remember Christine from the beginning of this chapter? She had a few extremely high adrenal cortisol levels. The problem with this is, what goes up, must come down. We can't predict when this will happen, but when it does, cortisol levels bottom out, causing additional and sometimes varied symptoms. The fact is, all women with hormonal imbalances have abnormal cortisol levels—some are high at times, and some are low.

Each adrenal gland is located above a kidney and contains an outer wall (the cortex) and an inner portion (the medulla). The adrenal glands converse nonstop with the posterior pituitary and the hypothalamus to maintain endocrine balance. They also elevate fatty acids and blood glucose, a.k.a. blood sugar, via the secretion of corticosteroids from the adrenal cortex. They affect protein breakdown and anti-inflammatory responses as well.

In women and men, some of the primary sex hormones testosterone and estrogen are manufactured in the adrenal glands. (You may not realize this, but even if you've had a complete hysterectomy, your body continues to secrete vital hormones, thanks to your adrenal glands. Your body is endowed with a hormone fail-safe, because Mother Nature empowers you to produce hormones as long as you live.)

Adrenal hormones perform many fascinating functions. Here's a condensed version of what these hormones are and do.

Glucocorticoids (certain steroids, cortisol, and corticosterone): Have various effects on inflammation and protein synthesis.

Mineralocorticoids (certain steroids; aldosterone): Maintain the body's salt balance.

Epinephrine (adrenaline): Regulates cardiac function, smooth muscle contraction, and the mobilization of fat cells.

Norepinephrine (noradrenaline): Facilitates fat cell mobilization and arteriole contraction.

Along with creating adrenaline, the adrenals produce cortisone-related hormones such as cortisol, the primary stress hormone, to control blood sugar. These hormones are chief players in the stress response, a complex mind/body state that most twenty-first-century women experience regularly. You'll learn more about the stress response and how to revitalize stressed hormones in chapter 5. In the meantime, consider the following facts on stress and hormones.

The stress response evolved over millions of years to help us efficiently fight opponents or run like the wind from threatening cavemen, landslides, and other terrors. When the stress response kicks in, adrenal hormones flow into your heart and raise your heart rate. This supplies more blood to move your muscles and activate your brain. Adrenal hormones also cause your blood vessels to constrict, which speeds up blood flow but can make you feel jittery, frightened, and cold in your hands and feet. It's the origin of the expression "cold feet."

During the stress response, cortisol flows freely with adrenaline. The main functions of adrenaline and cortisol include fueling fight-or-flight behavior during the stress response. Adrenaline also causes blood sugar to exit your liver, fat, and muscles, which gives your body more energy to meet physical and mental demands while under stress.

In addition to helping you function at peak efficiency during the stress response, cortisol promotes normal metabolism, maintains blood-sugar levels and blood pressure, and acts as an anti-inflammatory agent. Cortisol also helps to regulate the body's fluid balance.

On the down side, the primary stress hormone cortisol has many damaging effects that can make a huge difference to your hormone balance and, hence, your general well-being, brain function, and all hormonal symptoms. Before we go any further, here's a brief explanation of how cortisol and certain endocrine glands and hormones spring into action when you feel stressed.

The Cortisol Carousel: How This Stress Hormone Runs You Down
Cortisol can take your health and hormones on a wild ride. Along with being a marker of stress levels, cortisol is necessary for the functioning of almost every part of the body. It follows that cortisol excesses or deficiencies can lead to a wide range of physical symptoms and disease states. For example, abnormal cortisol levels are

documented cofactors in weight gain, increased appetite, diabetes, and depression. (You'll learn how elevated cortisol levels may affect your brain function and memory in chapter 5.)

Dozens of scientific studies confirm that the following three lifestyle traits contribute to abnormal cortisol levels: chronic stress (work deadlines, multiple family demands, financial problems, divorce, difficult marriage, commuting in traffic), sleeping less than eight hours each night, and restricting caloric intake for weight loss and dieting or maintaining strict limits on what you eat.

If you experience all three in your life, it's urgent that you make changes immediately. Even if just one applies to you, it's time to revamp your lifestyle and revitalize your hormones.

The guidelines in this book will show you how to create internal peace and balance your health so that your hormone levels return to normal.

When cortisol levels hit high peaks, the adrenal glands are too weak to make all the hormones that you need. This switches the pituitary gland into crisis mode, and a domino effect sweeps through your endocrine system, impairing glandular functions and causing one hormonal imbalance after another.

It's a scientific fact that chronic, excessive emotional stress, protein deficiency, and a lack of nutrients can exhaust the adrenal glands and render them incapable of producing adequate cortisol. Abnormal cortisol levels could fuel such symptoms as PMS, exhaustion, chronic irritability, and low energy. In chapter 5, you can take an Adrenal Stress Self-Assessment Test to learn more about adrenal cortisol and your health.

Any hormone guide must mention the lesser-known but mega-important calcitriol. This valiant substance is the kidney hormone, and it's responsible for maintaining the balance of calcium and phosphorus, increasing calcium uptake, and regulating bone mineralization. Then there is the cardiac hormone, atrial natriuretic peptide (ANP). It is released from the heart and acts on outer adrenal cells to decrease aldosterone production and promote smooth muscle relaxation.

How Stress Makes You Fat

Throughout history, humans have consumed high-fat or sugary comfort foods and alcohol, which is high in sugar, whenever they felt stressed or desired nurturing. As I've said for years, and as any nutritionist, psychologist, or physician will tell you, the behavioral response to stress can be a major cause of weight gain. But there are other body-based reasons for the link between stress and weight gain, and one of these is—surprise!—cortisol.

Whenever you're under stress, cortisol instant-messages your brain that you're hungry and you need to eat. This makes you reach for food even if your stomach is full. One awful truth about cortisol is that whenever you snack under stress, cortisol instructs your brain to program your fat cells to store fat! Stress always puts you in danger of gaining weight, because the more cortisol there is flowing through you, the more fat gets stored in your body.

Warning: When cortisol levels stay abnormal for prolonged periods, it's common for women to gain weight around the middle and the rear end. This is a compelling reason why you'll want to practice the stress-busting, hormone-revitalizing strategies in chapter 5.

Before you do that, however, here are some quick tips on how to avoid stress snacking. Never keep fattening foods in your home or office in the first place. Keep bottled spring water handy at all times, so that when you feel uptight and driven to snack, you can drink some pure water instead. Water fills you up, refreshes your body and mind, and helps you to defuse stress while you forget about food.

Another key point is that elevated cortisol can greatly affect your memory—or lack of it. When cortisol is released, it cripples the utilization of blood sugar by the brain's main memory center, the hippocampus. Blood sugar shortage means that the brain is energy-deprived and lacks the chemicals to create a clear and lasting memory. Unlike adrenaline, cortisol stays in your system much longer, and it steeps the brain in chemicals that injure and kill brain cells. Prolonged cortisol release can wipe out brain cells by the billions.

The Stress-Diabetes Connection

Having a genetic predisposition to diabetes is an important factor in whether you develop the condition. Yet stress, cortisol, and your pancreas also play pivotal roles. Diabetes is a chronic disease for which traditional medicine has no cure. It comes in two forms: type 1 diabetes (also known as juvenile diabetes) and type 2 diabetes, which develops in some children but is more common in adults (thus it's called "adult onset").

The American Diabetes Association's statistics show that diabetes is the sixth deadliest disease in the United States. In 2000, diabetes and its related complications claimed more than 213,000 lives. The total annual economic cost of diabetes in 2002 was a staggering $132 billion, or one out of every ten health-care dollars spent in the United States.

Of the estimated 18.2 million people with diabetes, 5.2 million remain unaware and undiagnosed. Diabetes is likely to be underreported as a cause of death because many descendants of people with diabetes do not have the disease entered on the death certificate. Studies have found that only about 35 to 40 percent have it listed anywhere on the certificate and only about 10 to 15 percent have it listed as the underlying cause of death. Overall, the risk for death among people with diabetes is about two times that of people without diabetes. Another 16 million Americans have impaired glucose tolerance (IGT) or pre-diabetes, a condition that is a precursor to type 2 adult onset diabetes. I mention this because many women who are, in fact, pre-diabetic present symptoms such as fatigue, depression, sugar cravings, overweight, and so on, which are often misdiagnosed or overlooked by doctors.

I have helped to facilitate the healing of pre-diabetes and diabetes with natural homeopathic remedies; vitamins and minerals; a balanced, low-carb, low-fat diet; and lifestyle changes, such as daily exercise that burns calories and fat. I believe that diabetes is curable, but to do so takes balancing the entire endocrine system using a multifaceted approach that includes energy medicine (homeopathy). The term *energy medicine* is commonly used among health-care providers who use homeopathy, electrodermal screening, electromagnetic field therapy, and advanced bioresonance medicine. Homeopathy is considered energy medicine because it has only the energy or memory of a substance in it. Moreover, balancing qi with qi gong and acupuncture is also referred to as energy medicine because acupuncture needles are inserted into energy channels.

If you think you might have either type of diabetes, the best way to find out is by consulting a holistic health-care provider. To diagnose diabetes, various tests are performed. A diabetic patient is typically diagnosed and monitored by measuring fasting blood glucose. This measurement, however, accurately reflects glucose concentrations only just prior to, and during, the collection time.

The Pancreas

In addition to the role that the pancreas plays in diabetes, it can affect your hormones in major ways. Consider the following, especially if you have PMS. The pancreas helps to control blood sugar levels. Blood sugar fluctuations can knock sex hormones for a loop, and unbalanced sex hormones can cause what you assume are menstrual problems. The real source of your problem, however, is not in your reproductive system but in your pancreas and the hormones it secretes.

Before we peer into pancreatic function, let's take a quick look at pancreatic hormones and what they do.

Insulin: Increases glucose uptake and utilization.

Glucagon: Increases fat cell mobilization and blood glucose levels.

Pancreatic polypeptide: Regulates gastrointestinal activity and other functions.

Somatostatin: Inhibits the release of glucagon and somatotropin (growth hormone), which are involved in numerous complex physiological processes.

The following scenario describes how you can develop what may be diagnosed as premenstrual syndrome or irritating perimenopausal symptoms. Your pancreas contains cells that secrete digestive enzymes into the small intestines and clusters of endocrine cells, which are called pancreatic islets.

The anatomical features of pancreatic islets in relation to hormone secretions and its control include approximately 1 million islets that constitute 1 to 1.5 percent of the total human pancreatic mass. The islets secrete the hormones insulin and glucagon, which regulate your blood sugar levels. After you eat, your blood sugar levels rise, triggering insulin release, which causes cells to take up glucose and liver and skeletal muscle cells to form the carbohydrate glycogen.

The higher your sugar intake, the more you abuse your pancreas, which is supposed to adjust insulin levels according to your needs.

The repeated insult of dealing with high and low sugar levels literally wears out the pancreas. As blood sugar levels fall, further insulin production is inhibited. This makes you feel draggy, weak, and tired—even more so before your period. Glucagon causes the breakdown of glycogen into sugar, which in turn is released into the bloodstream to maintain normal glucose (a.k.a. blood sugar levels). Glucagon production is stimulated when blood sugar levels fall and is inhibited when they rise.

Some people suffer from chronic low blood sugar, or hypoglycemia. This may be exacerbated by hormonal conditions, liver congestion, or pancreatic problems, or both. Maintaining a nutritious diet and avoiding sugar intake are key to having a healthy pancreas. The following Blood Sugar Self-Assessment Test will help you zero in on whether you may have hypoglycemia.

Blood Glucose Self-Assessment Test

Check off the symptoms that apply to you. Do you have . . . ?

- ☐ a craving for sweets or coffee in the afternoon or midmorning
- ☐ hunger between meals
- ☐ excessive appetite
- ☐ a tendency to eat when nervous
- ☐ irritability before meals
- ☐ shakiness or light-headedness while waiting for meals
- ☐ heart palpitations if meals are missed or delayed
- ☐ fatigue that is relieved by eating
- ☐ wakefulness a few hours after going to sleep
- ☐ difficulty falling back asleep
- ☐ sluggishness; fatigue
- ☐ lethargy; apathy
- ☐ hyperactivity
- ☐ restlessness
- ☐ mood swings
- ☐ anxiety, fear, or nervousness
- ☐ depression
- ☐ poor memory
- ☐ confusion; poor comprehension
- ☐ poor concentration
- ☐ poor physical condition
- ☐ difficulty making decisions
- ☐ stuttering or stammering
- ☐ slurred speech
- ☐ learning disabilities

☐ binge eating   ☐ compulsive eating
☐ binge drinking   ☐ water retention
☐ food cravings   ☐ underweight
☐ excessive weight   ☐ hot flashes

If you've checked four or more symptoms and suspect that you may have hypoglycemia, you might want to try following a sugar-free, low-carb diet, because carbs convert into sugar inside the body. (See the recommendations for natural sugar substitutes in chapter 4.) Or, you may benefit from taking nutritional supplements such as chromium picolinate with boron, which has been shown in studies to help normalize blood sugar.

The most accurate way to diagnose low blood sugar is with an eight-hour fasting glucose test, which any clinical laboratory can do for you.

At this point in our hormone tour, we need to scope out the various hormones that promote the complex chemical process of digestion. Many people are amazed when I tell them that our bodies contain digestive hormones that help us absorb nutrients from food. Here is an overview:

Gastrin: Stimulates acid, pepsin, and pancreatic secretions.

Secretin: Stimulates pancreatic cells to release water and other essential substances.

Cholecystokinin (CCK): Stimulates gallbladder contraction and bile flow; increases the secretion of digestive enzymes from the pancreas.

Motilin: Controls the gastrointestinal (GI) muscles.

Vasoactive intestinal peptide (VIP): Relaxes the GI tract; inhibits acid and pepsin secretion; acts as a neurotransmitter in smooth muscle relaxation and enhances genital blood flow during sexual arousal; increases the secretion of water and electrolytes from the pancreas and the gut.

Gastric inhibitory peptide (GIP): Inhibits the secretion of gastrin.

Somatostatin: Inhibits gastrin secretion from the stomach and glucagon secretion from the pancreas.

The Liver

The next stop on our endocrine odyssey is the liver. The liver performs many heroic tasks, including the conjugation of hormones. The liver hormone angiotensin II is responsible for releasing the hormone aldosterone from adrenal cells. If your liver is burdened with environmental chemicals, prescription medications, or recreational drugs, you may have hormone imbalances due to liver toxicity. In chapter 3, you'll find several methods for detoxifying the body and its filtering organs, such as the liver and the kidneys.

The Ovaries

Two of the most crucial endocrine glands are the ovaries. Located on the right and the left sides of your pelvis about two inches below the navel, the ovaries produce essential sex hormones that make you feel, look, walk, and talk like a woman. The main hormones produced by the ovaries are

Estrogen steroids, which include estradiol, estrone, and estriol: Produced by the adrenal glands for as long as you live, *estradiol* activates growth of the breasts and other female sex organs. It also promotes the maturation of long bones and the development of secondary sexual characteristics. Unbalanced estrogen levels can cause urinary incontinence in women who are experiencing perimenopause, menopause, or extreme endocrine breakdown.

Estrone: Produced primarily from androstenodione that originates in the ovaries or the adrenal cortex. In premenopausal women, more than 50 percent of estrone is secreted by the ovaries. In premenopausal women, estrone levels generally parallel those of estradiol. After menopause, estrone levels increase, perhaps because of the increased conversion of androstenodione to estrone.

Estriol: This plays a vital role in the health of the female reproductive organs and is the estrogen that is most beneficial to the vagina and the cervical tissue. Estriol is produced in large quantities (with progesterone) during pregnancy. High levels of estriol have been found in Asian women, who consistently appear to be at much lower risk of contracting breast cancer than are American women. In animal studies, it appears that estriol is less carcinogenic than estradiol and estrone are. Research has demonstrated that women with breast cancer have a reduced excretion of estriol, as compared to healthy women.

Progesterone: Assists in egg implantation and helps to maintain pregnancy.

Testosterone: Is critical to women's hormonal and sexual health, energy levels, and mood. When the ovaries shut down at menopause, the amount of testosterone they produce is reduced by half. For many women, this results in diminished sexual desire, thinning pubic hair, flatness of mood, dry skin, and decreased mental sharpness, among other symptoms.

Intimately involved in stoking female libido, arousal, and achieving orgasm, testosterone also helps to promote a sense of well-being. Research indicates that testosterone strongly influences female behavior and can even confer more social power on women who have comparatively higher levels of it.

A recent study by Dr. Valerie Grant at the University of Auckland, New Zealand, found that a woman's relative dominance is strongly linked to how high her testosterone levels are. A previous similar study found much higher testosterone levels in professional and managerial women than in housewives and clerical workers.

Testosterone replacement therapy is even making headlines as a trendy hormone replacement cocktail among certain female political leaders. A leading London gynecologist, Dr. Malcolm Whitehead, told the British magazine the *New Statesman* that he is increasingly prescribing testosterone implants for women members of parliament. "I have prescribed testosterone implants for female politicians in Westminster who want to compete better with their male colleagues in committee meetings and parliamentary debates," said Dr. Whitehead. "They claim the hormone boosts their assertiveness and makes them feel more powerful." Hmm. I hope they're also enjoying enhanced libido and more dynamic orgasms, thanks to all that testosterone.

Anyone who takes testosterone supplements needs to be

careful. Side effects of testosterone toxicity may include facial and body hair growth, voice deepening, bouts of anger and rage, depression, increased muscle mass, menstrual interruption, and, of course, hormonal imbalance.

The female members of parliament highlight how important testosterone can be to female confidence, professional success, and social stature. I know, from my private practice and from reviewing thousands of before-and-after saliva tests, that many women are misdiagnosed as depressed and are prescribed anti-depressants when they simply need natural endocrine revitalization to remedy low testosterone levels. In the following chapters, you'll learn how to help your body make its own testosterone.

The Uterus and Endometriosis

The uterus is an ingenious endocrine gland. It is our first home, the nurturing environment for a growing baby. The health and the function of the uterus are greatly influenced by hormonal health. Let's take a look at endometriosis now, because it has been clearly documented that unbalanced hormones are a prime cause of this chronic, painful, and often misdiagnosed uterine-related condition.

It is reported that endometriosis afflicts at least one in seven women. The disease occurs when uterine lining tissue (the endometrium) is found outside the uterus, usually in the abdomen or on the ovaries, the fallopian tubes, and the ligaments that support the uterus. Tissue may also be found in the area between the vagina and the rectum, on the outer surface of the uterus, and in the lining of the pelvic cavity.

Other sites for endometrial growths may include the bladder, the bowel, the vagina, the cervix, the vulva, and inside abdominal surgical scars. Less commonly, they are found in the lungs, the arms, the thighs, and other locations. This misplaced tissue develops into growths or lesions that respond to the menstrual cycle in the same way that the tissue of the uterine lining does: each month the tissue builds up, breaks down, and sheds.

Menstrual blood flows from the uterus and out of the body through the vagina, but the blood and tissue that's shed from endometrial growths has no way of leaving the body. This results in internal bleeding, breakdown of the blood and the tissue from the lesions, and inflammation. It can cause pain, infertility, scar tissue formation, adhesions, and bowel problems. Diagnosis is considered uncertain until proven by laparoscopy, a minor surgical procedure done under anesthesia. A laparoscopy usually shows the location, the size, and the extent of the growths. This helps the doctor and the patient make better treatment choices.

Endometriosis can strike a woman when she is still in her teens. Symptoms resemble those of many other illnesses, and women with endometriosis appear perfectly well. Because of these factors, endometriosis often goes undiagnosed. It's quite possible that many more than 10 percent of women in the general population may have it. Every woman should understand the basics about endometriosis to gain insight into how our bodies work and what we can do to keep ourselves healthy. Take, for example, the story of my patient Carrie, who was only twenty-six when she sought my help.

I've had endometriosis for six years. I underwent laparoscopic surgery a year ago, but it returned months later after I stopped getting monthly Lupron injections. I tried Depo-Provera but had some complications with it. My ob/gyn now has me on the birth control pill Levlen 28 on a noncyclic basis (skipping the placebos and starting a new pack). Is this really a reasonable treatment? I'm worried that never having a period is unhealthy. I don't plan on having children for at least another two years.

Continuous use of oral contraceptives is a well-known treatment that suppresses endometriosis without curing it. Treating a hormonal-related problem with synthetic hormones serves only to stress the adrenal glands and create additional hormone disturbances. Carrie was right to question how taking hormones and never menstruating might affect her health. I gave her homeopathic remedies, as well as a nutritional regimen that is discussed in chapter 4. After a few months, Carrie's pelvic pain lessened dramatically, her periods resumed, and the endometriosis stopped.

I invite you to take the following self-assessment test to see if some of your symptoms resemble those of endometriosis. Warning: This is a difficult diagnosis. Symptoms such as menstrual pain, bloating, pain with sex, or pelvic discomfort, from ovulation to the time of your period, heighten the index of suspicion but aren't conclusive. While some women have the condition but never exhibit symptoms, others have symptoms but no endometriosis. The amount of pain a woman may experience isn't related to the number or the size of her endometrial growths. Some women with moderate to severe endometriosis have no pain, while others with a minor condition experience severe pain.

If you have two or more of these symptoms, I urge you to see a holistic health practitioner and try the nutritional and homeopathic strategies detailed in this book.

Endometriosis Self-Assessment Test

Check off the symptoms that apply to you.

☐ chronic pelvic pain

☐ pain before menstruation (dysmenorrhea)

☐ pain during menstruation (dysmenorrhea)

☐ pain during and after sexual intercourse (dyspareunia)

☐ irregular vaginal bleeding

☐ infertility

☐ painful bowel movements during menstruation

☐ fatigue

☐ abdominal bloating

Along with their contributing role in endometriosis, hormonal imbalances are intimately connected to the development of uterine fibroids. Hysterectomy, or the surgical removal of the ovaries and the uterus, is known to trigger hormone deficiencies, causing an array of uncomfortable symptoms that are usually treated with conventional or so-called natural HRT. To complete our discussion of the uterus, let's take a look at the complex issues related to hysterectomy.

Hysterectomy

This happens to be the second-most common major operation performed on women. Various forms of HRT are routinely prescribed to women after hysterectomy. There is widespread concern among researchers and the public that hysterectomy may be extremely overused. Recent authoritative research strongly suggests this may be the case.

According to a study published in the peer-reviewed medical

journal *Obstetrics & Gynecology*, "As many as 70 percent of hysterectomies performed in the US may be recommended inappropriately. . . . We found that the care leading to recommendations of hysterectomies in our cohort was sub-optimal." Yes, you read that correctly: as many as 70 percent of all hysterectomies performed in the United States may be unnecessary. Statistics like these are further reminders that all women must take primary responsibility for their hormonal and reproductive health care.

The researchers tracked about five hundred women who had hysterectomies that were not due to cancer or an emergency. (The operations were performed over a two-year period in Southern California.) Investigators found that many of the women never received adequate evaluations of the potential causes of their medical problems—for example, a laparoscopy to help determine the cause of pelvic pain, a hormone saliva test to assess hormone levels, or a sampling of the uterine lining to determine the cause of abnormal bleeding.

Many women also failed to try alternative, evidence-based natural therapies, such as nutrition, herbs, or homeopathy, before their surgery. Sixty percent of hysterectomies were recommended due to fibroids (benign tumors that commonly occur in middle-aged women), 11 percent due to pelvic relaxation, 9 percent due to pain, and 8 percent due to bleeding.

These alarming findings are a stark warning that we should always investigate the potential causes of symptoms such as pain or bleeding. Women must explore natural remedies and treatment methods with a holistic health-care provider before they resort to having a hysterectomy.

Now that we've toured the endocrine system and know its key glands and hormones, let's consider the documented causes of endocrine breakdown, which can generate so many uncomfortable symptoms. (Chapter 7 contains homeopathic remedies to detoxify the body of substances that are involved in endocrine breakdown.) Let me start by saying that your genetics play a role in your overall health. Genetic predispositions to disease can be overcome to a great degree through making a lifestyle change and using natural therapies. Moreover, I have clarified nine additional causes of endocrine breakdown.

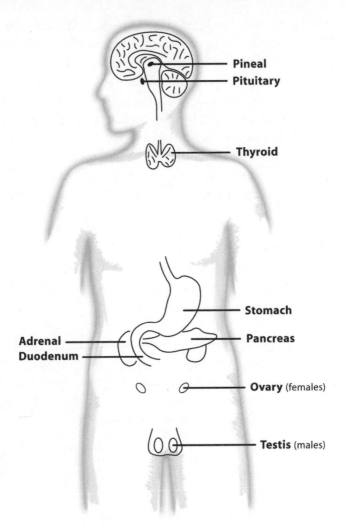

Pineal
Pituitary

Thyroid

Stomach

Adrenal
Duodenum

Pancreas

Ovary (females)

Testis (males)

FIGURE 1: THE ENDOCRINE SYSTEM

The Nine Causes of Endocrine Breakdown

1. *Weakened immunity*. Lyme disease, viruses, bacteria, herpes, mononucleosis, impaired immune function, and any pathology that impairs adrenal function can seriously compromise the endocrine system. Whenever the immune system is weakened, viruses, bacteria, microbes, or parasites find it easiest to invade and occupy the body. The good news is that you can strengthen your immune system. Strategies for doing this are given throughout the book.

2. *Dental conditions.* Abscesses, infections, and root canals on endocrine acupuncture meridians that flow through teeth can impair endocrine function. Evidence strongly suggests that mercury toxicity can damage the endocrine system and other parts of the body as well. Mercury can cross the blood-brain barrier, thus impairing pituitary and hypothalamus functions. To detoxify mercury or other heavy metals from your body, you can use the homeopathic remedies in chapter 7, as well as take special vitamin C ascorbate with MSM.

   In the United States and elsewhere, many physicians and naturopathic doctors consider mercury toxicity a potent underlying cause of chronic illness. Some of these doctors refuse to take on new patients who have mercury fillings and root canals until these are removed by a holistic dentist and refilled with a biocompatible substance for your body, which is determined by blood testing. (You'll find information on holistic dentists in your area in the Resource Guide.)

3. *Imbalanced autonomic nervous system.* The balance of the autonomic nervous system (ANS), or sympathetic/parasympathetic nervous system, is key to maintaining healthy endocrine function. It's important to understand the ANS because it controls many organs, including the endocrine glands, which secrete your hormones.

   The sympathetic nervous system has many fascinating powers, such as orchestrating sexual arousal and preparing the body for action by speeding up the heart rate. While the sympathetic nervous system functions rather like the fast-forward mechanism on a DVD player, the parasympathetic nervous system functions similarly to the pause button.

   Here's an example of how the two zones spring into action. When we exercise, the sympathetic nervous system jacks up the heart rate. When we stretch and cool off afterward, the parasympathetic helps to slow the heart rate way down, which in turn slows down brain waves. This initiates the relaxation response and a release of feel-good hormones like endorphins, which in turn promotes calm and heightened immunity. Chiropractic care can help to promote healthy autonomic nervous system function.

4. *Neurotransmitter imbalances.* Neurotransmitters are the chemical messengers that relay signals between nerve cells. Imbalances in neurotransmitters can cause weight gain, insomnia, weight loss, depression, anxiety, fatigue, memory loss, mood swings, and ADD or ADHD. Constructed from amino acids, vitamins, and mineral cofactors within the body, neurotransmitters critically support autonomic nervous system functions and strongly influence moods, behavior, cognitive processes, social attitudes, digestion, and sleep. Certain neurotransmitters even control smooth muscle relaxation and enhance genital blood flow during lovemaking.

   Neurotransmitters control your ability to feel, think, and experience emotions. If the body lacks a sufficient supply of neurotransmitters, depletion occurs, which leads to inadequate neurotransmission with systemic results; in other words, your hormone levels will be negatively affected.

   For instance, the neurotransmitter dopamine stimulates the release of the hormone oxytocin. Oxytocin promotes sexual arousal, feelings of emotional attachment, and the desire to cuddle; it also stimulates milk secretion when nursing. I've met with women who believed they were suffering from sexual dysfunction and depression. After I conducted tests on them, you can imagine their relief when I revealed that they merely had a dopamine deficiency.

   It's entirely possible that neurotransmitter imbalances affect a significant portion of the population. Research indicates that some neurotransmitters are negatively affected by toxins such as mercury, which is commonly found in dental amalgam fillings, shark, tuna, and other fish.

   Deficiencies in the neurotransmitter serotonin can cause depression and can initiate the stress response, triggering the release of stress hormones. This makes you feel even more depressed and self-doubting and sets up a vicious cycle. (You'll learn more about neurotransmitters and their relationship to stress levels in chapter 5, as well as several effective stress-reduction strategies that you can practice immediately.

5. *Imbalanced diet and lifestyle.* If your diet consists of processed, chemically laden, dead foods that are high in toxins (such as partially hydrogenated oils), which make you overweight, and you

rarely exercise, this can negatively affect your endocrine system. Obesity is a marker of many underlying health and lifestyle problems.

Consuming large quantities of alcohol, caffeine, and food preservatives on a daily basis can also undermine endocrine functioning. While thyroid and adrenal problems can put you in the firing line for obesity, the trigger is pulled by diet and lifestyle. Unfortunately, thyroid treatments that fail to simultaneously support adrenal gland functions can contribute to endocrine breakdown as well.

Eating disorders also seriously strain the endocrine glands and have a negative effect on hormone balance. This is one reason why many women with eating disorders have irregular menstrual periods or no periods at all.

6. *Emotional issues.* While regular caffeine consumption and recreational drug use can trigger adrenal stress, emotional burnout and psychological trauma can also heavily tax the adrenal glands and create hormonal crises. Persuasive research indicates that relationship and career-related stress, along with repressed and unresolved childhood emotional issues, can stress all organs and glands. Please see the Five Element Body Clock on page 62 and chapter 6 for details on emotional connection.

Several decades ago, the noted stress researcher Hans Selye proved that even positive emotional events, like moving into your dream house or starting a new job, can stress the body by exerting wear and tear on organs and body systems. You may have heard of psychoneuroimmunology (PNI). This branch of medicine investigates the links between psychological states and immune system functioning, and how our minds and emotions can suppress or bolster immune function. PNI research has yielded many insights into how psychological states affect resistance or vulnerability to disease. It's been proved that negative emotions burden the immune system, thus adversely affecting adrenal cortisol levels and other endocrine functions.

7. *Scar tissue.* If scar tissue is located over an acupuncture endocrine meridian, it can block the flow of electromagnetic energy through organs and body systems. This may suppress endocrine system feedback mechanisms, causing hormone levels to fall out of proper balance.

8. *Medications.* Hormone replacement therapy (HRT) of any kind (including natural and bio-identical) is a source of endocrine breakdown for all the reasons noted in this book. Most medications have a negative effect on the body; some examples are cortisone, anti-inflammatory drugs, glucose regulating drugs such as insulin, thyroid regulating drugs, antibiotics, and high blood pressure medications.

9. *Environmental toxins.* In addition to hormone-disrupting agricultural, plastic, cosmetic, and household cleaner products that I'll detail later in this chapter, there are several other environmental causes of endocrine breakdown. These include electromagnetic fields (EMFs) and radio frequency fields (RFs).

   I benefit from twenty-first-century technologies as much as the next person, but I must tell you that the RFs produced by computer monitors, microwave ovens, and cellular telephones are classified by the World Health Organization, the National Institute of Environmental Health Sciences (NIEHS), and other scientific authorities as 2B, or "possible carcinogens." (To put this in perspective, DDT and lead are also classified as 2B carcinogens. It's well documented that these may cause birth defects, brain damage, cancers, and a host of other serious illnesses.)

   A mounting body of evidence suggests that the RFs generated by cell phones may adversely affect health. Radio frequency waves generated by wireless technologies are becoming increasingly urgent health concerns, because these are known to adversely affect the autonomic nervous system and disrupt endocrine functions and therefore reproductive development. (I use a cell phone, but with an earpiece attachment, so that I don't have to hold it to my head.)

   Research scientists like Cindy Sage of Sage Associates in Santa Barbara, California, use computer modeling to estimate how children and adults may be negatively affected by radio frequencies. "A large body of evidence indicates that children under the age of 16 should not use mobile phones because their nervous and reproductive systems are still developing and their skulls are thinner than adult skulls."

   Research has proved that RF exposure adversely affects hormones, says Cindy Sage. For example, she notes, "Sleeping in the midst of RF fields throws cortisol profiles off."

Furthermore, some research shows that single- and double-strand DNA damage results from radio frequency exposures that are well under the federal limits. "While microwatt RF may be under the federal limits, this is still enough to deregulate all major circadian rhythms and body systems, including the endocrine system and its hormones," Sage says. This last warning is especially applicable to people who frequently use a cell phone, a Blackberry, a wireless computer, or all three.

Other environmental risks to hormone health include living near microwave towers. Some evidence also indicates that using electric blankets or having televisions, stereos, or other electrical equipment within four feet of your bed may pose health risks. Certain studies suggest that sleeping in a bedroom that has water pipes underneath it, or living above an underground stream, may also expose you to potentially dangerous electromagnetic fields.

A patient of mine, a highly driven attorney, used her cell phone six to eight hours per day. She told me that she often felt flooded with intense emotions and experienced continual burning sensations, along with an ache inside her head on the right side where she always held the cell phone. During an NPR session, I discovered that her right ear and her mastoid gland tested as being inflamed and weak.

Since I was uncertain whether her symptoms were developing into a tumor or a cyst, I immediately recommended that she suspend cell phone use for one month so that she could feel whether it made a difference. In addition, I suggested that she incorporate a homeopathic remedy for detoxifying radiation into her program and that if the symptoms persisted after one month, she should get an MRI. After two weeks, she reported that the physical burning and the ache had faded by 50 percent, and the next month all symptoms disappeared.

Hormones in Our Food, Water, Household Products, and Environment

Research has conclusively proved that American women have the highest levels of estrogen in the world. Wow! This excess probably comes from xenoestrogens (which literally means "foreign estrogens") in our food, household products, and environment.

Xenoestrogens are compounds whose molecular structure is so similar to estrogen that they have estrogenic effects in the body. Xenoestrogens are classed as endocrine-disrupting chemicals (EDCs). This is because they disrupt hormone balance and endocrine system functioning, thus increasing the risk of cancer and other diseases.

Endocrine-disrupting compounds include

growth hormones used in milk, cheese, and meat production. (Few nutritionally oriented doctors mention the importance of eating organic meat and dairy foods, to avoid the dangers of consuming growth hormones. You'll learn more about the health and beauty benefits of eating organically in chapter 4 and will find delicious recipes in part 3.)

chemicals such as PCBs, found in freshwater and saltwater fish

chemicals such as organochlorines, thousands of which are in our water supply and are thus ingested every day when we bathe, brush our teeth, or drink tap water

agricultural pesticides, which are sprayed on all conventionally grown fruits, vegetables, grains, nuts, and herbs, but never on organically grown foods

chemicals found in color cosmetics, hair dyes, and skin care products

chemicals released by plastic wraps and food containers when they're heated in microwaves

chemicals in hard plastic toys

chemicals found in household cleaning products and detergents

As I mentioned previously, estrogen's natural function is to stimulate cell growth. But excess estrogen contributes to unnatural growth, and therein lies the danger. A 2003 study by the Harvard University School of Public Health and the Silent Spring Institute in Newton, Massachusetts, discovered that several toxic, hormone-altering chemical compounds that are rarely listed as ingredients in detergents and cleaning products had poisoned the indoor air and the dust of 120 homes in residential areas.

While the study didn't examine whether people within the households had actually ingested or inhaled the chemicals from the dust and the indoor air, a previous study by the U.S. Centers for Disease Control and Prevention found many of the same chemicals inside the bodies of Americans. Although there is a hormonal component to most cancers, estrogen dominance has been documented as playing a leading role in breast, uterine, and ovarian cancers.

The Harvard/Silent Spring study demonstrated that we're exposed daily to a wide array of chemicals that affects our hormone systems. Nine chemical compounds were found in every house tested. Six are phthalates, found mostly in cosmetics and hard plastics, and three are alkylphenols, including one that's commonly used in detergents and cleansers.

Please note that women of childbearing age and children are considered at highest risk to hormone-altering compounds because exposure may damage the sexual and neurological development of fetuses and growing children. While some scientists theorize that endocrine disrupters may also heighten the risk of hormonal diseases, including testicular and breast cancer, the full extent of health risks posed by hormone-altering compounds remains unknown.

The best way to limit your exposure is to read labels carefully, use nontoxic cleaning products, and avoid using indoor pesticides, which also contain endocrine disrupters.

It's essential to understand that many EDCs are in our water. Every time you drink tap water or bathe, you ingest or inhale the toxic chemical chlorine and other substances that it combines with in water to create toxic by-products called organochlorines. These by-products are present in more than 96 percent of agricultural chemicals.

Organochlorines include EDCs, such as PCBs, dioxins, and the pesticide DDT. There is some evidence that EDCs contribute to breast, prostate, testicular, and other cancers. As long ago as 1964, the World Health Organization reported that 80 percent of cancers were due to industrial carcinogens like EDCs.

For most carcinogens, a minimum exposure is necessary for a person to develop cancer. Even when individuals are exposed to the same carcinogens, they exhibit varying susceptibilities to developing cancer, based upon genetic makeup and individual health.

Regarding other toxins in our water, the EPA Web site notes that fuel additives have leached through storage tanks into every municipal water supply in the country. I hate to bring more bad news, but high amounts of arsenic, fluoride, nickel, and other heavy metals are also present in our water. In addition, many studies have found that water pipes around the country harbor legionella (the bacterium also known as Legionnaires' Disease), plus parasites and other mysterious microbes.

Even purportedly pure bottled water must be checked for toxins. Read the labels first before buying. You may be surprised to find what chemicals are listed there! I know I have been.

Tuna, shark, and swordfish contain dangerously high mercury levels, due to oceanic pollution. Recent U.S. government and independent research advisories have cautioned that pregnant women and children should eliminate all tuna, shark, and swordfish from their diets. Other toxins found in the fatty tissues of marine animals such as fish, whales, and sharks are endocrine-disrupting PCBs, or polychlorinated biphenyls.

Here are the ABCs of PCBs. This group of compounds was developed in the 1930s and mainly used in the mining and electricity supply industries. PCBs are extremely stable, long-lasting chemicals. Although they were outlawed in Europe at the beginning of the 1980s, the United States only got around to banning them in 1997. PCBs are inside fish, sharks, whales, and marine birds. I love fish and don't want to bring you down, but PCBs have been found in some of the favorite foods of health-conscious people, such as Alaskan wild salmon.

In both humans and animals, PCB exposure has been scientifically linked with developmental and reproductive abnormalities, endocrine disruption, neurological dysfunction, and compromised immune systems. (In case you wonder how I've authenticated this information, its source happens to be the U.S. government's Environmental Protection Agency [EPA] Web site, www.epa.gov.)

For the developing fetus and the growing child, the harm of PCB exposure is the greatest. Because PCBs are stored in fat, they pass from the mother to the fetus during pregnancy, the most critical period of human development. For the developing infant, PCBs then pass through breast milk to be absorbed and stored in the growing child's body. Because of the serious hormonal and other health risks associated with PCBs, I advise that you limit your intake of all seafood.

On the brighter side, in chapter 3 you'll find an easy-to-follow guide to cutting endocrine disrupters out of your life.

Charting Your Hormonal Symptoms

More than twenty-three centuries before Western laboratory scientists invented HRT in an attempt to remedy hormonal-related conditions, Chinese Five Element Theory treated PMS, postpartum depression, and perimenopausal and postmenopausal problems with comprehensive diagnosis, acupuncture, massage, customized Chinese herbal tea remedies, and more.

Chinese herbal remedies are effective, and I use them in many situations. Unlike homeopathic hormone revitalization, however, Chinese herbs must be taken continuously for the individual to benefit. With homeopathy, you can achieve long-term results within a limited time frame. Homeopathic remedies are never taken over the long term.

The ancient Chinese worldview defined human beings as microcosms of the universe that surrounded them and assumed that they were influenced by the same elemental energies that powered the macrocosm. As profoundly holistic thinkers, the Chinese further defined themselves as part of one seamless wholeness, called Tao, a unified, all-inclusive, eternal continuum within and without. The Taoist conception of existence is the opposite of the mind/body split that Western philosophers dictated in the seventeenth century—and Western civilization has widened that gap ever since. Furthermore, the Taoist worldview is the opposite of the Western philosophical notion that humanity is autonomous and therefore removed from nature.

TCM sees the patient as living within a specific natural environment and treats people with nature-based plant and other healing remedies that are appropriate to each patient's environment, climate, and personal circumstances at the time of diagnosis. Ancient Chinese physicians were astute, methodical observers and diagnosticians. All examinations were done with their patients fully clothed. Doctors took pulses in both wrists and at the neck and noted with extreme interest the exact times of day when their patients' symptoms were most intense. This is because the doctors had discovered that symptoms that occurred repeatedly at any given time pointed to a problem in a particular body area.

One formal result of these observations is the Chinese Body Clock, which has been used for millennia to help diagnose patients. (See the figure on page 62.)

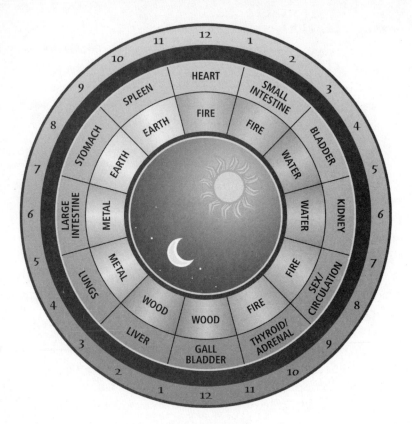

FIGURE 2: FIVE ELEMENT BODY CLOCK

As you can see, each two-hour time period corresponds to a particular part of the body. By using the Chinese Body Clock to record how you feel throughout the twenty-four-hour cycle, in conjunction with the principles of modern naturopathic medicine, you can identify which part of your hormonal system is the root cause of your symptoms. Another integral aspect of traditional Chinese medicine (TCM) is the Five Element Theory.

TCM considers the Five Elements of fire, earth, water, metal, and wood to be the foundation of all healing. Each part of your body, your emotional life, and even the food you eat belongs to one of the Five Elements, and the Chinese Body Clock relates each element to a specific time of day. The following chart is excerpted from the body clock figure and shows examples of the times of day that correspond to various organs and elements.

Time	Organ/Body Function	Element
8:00 A.M.	stomach	earth
10:00 A.M.	spleen	earth
Noon	heart	fire
2:00 P.M.	small intestine	fire
4:00 P.M.	bladder	water
6:00 P.M.	kidney	water
8:00 P.M.	sex/circulation meridian	fire
10:00 P.M.	thyroid/adrenal	fire
Midnight	gallbladder	wood
2:00 A.M.	liver	wood
4:00 A.M.	lungs	metal
6:00 A.M.	large intestine	metal

The Chinese Body Clock gives you the point of departure to find which organ is out of balance, but if you're like most people with hormone problems, you may have several organs out of balance and several times of day when your symptoms worsen. It can be confusing to know where to begin, but I'll help you.

It's easy to start. Simply take five sheets of paper and write down each hour from 1:00 A.M. to midnight. Every day, write down your symptoms at the exact time they occur, and rate their severity from mild to moderate to heavy. Now check to see the times that they're worse and whether they recur at the same time each day. You're looking for a regular time pattern to your symptoms. Once you identify which element(s) are out of balance, you'll be able to get to the root cause of your symptoms.

For example, if you have symptoms that manifest at 2:00 A.M. and 8 A.M., this indicates problems in the liver and the stomach. To begin with, you may benefit from detoxifying the liver (strategies for this are in chapter 3) and from eating foods that support liver function, while avoiding those that stress it, such as hot spicy foods and alcohol. Homeopathic remedies for supporting liver function are found in chapter 7's homeopathic chart. (You'll find homeopathic remedies for all other organs as well in the same chapter.)

Regarding your stomach issues, you may also benefit from eating foods that support digestion. These are discussed in chapters 3 and 4. I encourage you to note your symptoms and connect the dots to your organs by using the Chinese Body Clock, not just once, but every three months or so. Seasonal changes can affect your symptoms and can change your hormone levels in subtle, yet profound, ways.

Knowing why your hormones are out of balance is critical to permanently correcting them. Now that you've learned about some of your most influential hormones, I hope you realize what a worthwhile and monumental task it is to revitalize them.

I've said it before and I'll say it again: the goal of hormone revitalization is to make your own hormones, and you can do this with self-nurturing, detoxification, a good diet, and lifestyle support. You now know the hormone basics; the next step is to detoxify your body so that your endocrine system is strong enough to make your own hormones. You're in for a transforming experience, for the detoxification process will make your body and mind feel stronger, steadier, and calmer.

Step 2 Action Plan

1. If you haven't done so already, take all of the self-assessment tests in this chapter to get a clearer picture of your endocrine and hormonal health.
2. Do the Five Element Self-Diagnosis and write down the results.
3. Begin to rebalance your hormones by eliminating farmed fish from your diet, along with conventional meats and dairy products, which contain growth hormones.
4. Write down all of your physical and mental health symptoms, and use them as part of your Five Element Self-Diagnosis. Refer to these as you continue through the 7-Step Program.

Part Two

The Program to Heal, Strengthen, and Revitalize Your Body and Hormones

Step 3

Starting Fresh with Detoxification

At forty-six, Elizabeth was twenty pounds overweight and had an ash-gray complexion. She looked and acted older than her years. She was referred to me by her physician, who had been unable to remedy her physical and mental perimenopausal symptoms. (The "natural" progesterone cream she had been using seemed to have no effect on her anxiety, insomnia, weight problems, and bloating.) A perfectly pleasant woman, Elizabeth still struck me as anxious and upset. Her fidgety, tense movements expressed considerable inner turmoil. Elizabeth tried to mask her emotions with a big smile that telegraphed: "Help, I feel miserable, but I am determined to soldier through!"

Saliva tests indicated that Elizabeth's hormone levels were extremely out of balance. Her progesterone soared into the stratosphere and her DHEA levels registered in the deep end. What most alarmed me, though, was her appearance. She looked closer to sixty than to forty-six. As I do with all my patients, I gave Elizabeth a comprehensive biological age questionnaire. (Biological age is an estimate of how healthy you are, rather than a statement of your chronological age.)

The biological age questionnaire is a detailed inquiry into health history, eating habits, exercise, and lifestyle. As we reviewed her answers together, I connected Elizabeth's irritating symptoms and her appearance with toxic chemicals in the foods and the drinks she consumed, chemicals in her home environment, and the drugs she'd been taking, such as progesterone.

Elizabeth agreed, as does everyone I work with, that cleaning up her body would most likely make her feel better. Detoxifying her body and her environment, as well as detoxifying through daily exercise, represented a logical and effective step that would help her body produce appropriate amounts of hormones on a regular basis.

Toward that end, she immediately ceased taking drugs, including the so-called natural progesterone. She switched from chemically laden processed foods to eating as organically as her budget and schedule allowed. Along with installing air purifiers in her living room and bedroom, Elizabeth put water filters on her faucets and shower head to remove toxins like chlorine and bacteria from her drinking and bath water. Within six weeks, Elizabeth reported feeling calmer, yet much more energetic. I was happy to see that her skin looked brighter and her body trimmer. Patients like Elizabeth inspire me because they prove that living naturally can purify the body and renew the mind and spirit.

This chapter contains inspiration, along with information, to help you live a healthful life. As you'll see, the story of how biological age and toxins are interrelated is actually quite compelling. In the following pages, you'll learn how you can influence the rate at which you age, depending on how nontoxic your home and work environments are, the quality of your diet, how much you exercise, and how you manage your health. You'll also be given action plans to reduce your biological age by detoxifying so that you can make the hormones you need to feel and look younger, sexier, and stronger. Before we go any further into detoxification, though, it's helpful to understand the fundamental causes of aging.

The Art and the Science of Antiaging

Three main factors contribute to aging: aging of the cardiovascular system, aging of the immune system, and aging caused by accidents and environmental factors. Arterial aging is the root cause of heart attacks, strokes, heart disease, and even Alzheimer's disease.

Immune system aging is associated with cancers and autoimmune diseases such as arthritis. Although many people believe that cardio-vascular disease and cancer are caused by genetics or bad luck, the truth is that 70 percent of arterial aging is preventable. And 80 to 90 percent of all cancers are due to HRT and/or environmental causes, such as exposure to toxins, poor diet, a sedentary lifestyle, prolonged stress, or a combination of all four.

How do you know if you are relatively toxin-free? Complete the following Biological Age Assessment Quiz (see page 70). Biological age refers to the age of your organs and how toxic or healthy they are. The quiz helps you to approximate your real age. Once you have finished, add and subtract the points corresponding to your answers from your current chronological age. This will give you an approximation of your biological age and also recommendations for correcting a high biological age.

Now that you know your biological age, you also have an outline of which foods, drugs, and environmental factors shape your health history and your present state. Some of these foods, drugs, and factors are toxins.

Detoxifying Your Habits

While you learn how to effectively detoxify your body and treat common toxicity and hormone-related problems, it's essential to recognize that the toxins you are exposed to each day can be decreased through new choices.

The Air You Breathe

The toxins that you ingest through outdoor air pollution contribute to the aging process, as do the toxins in your indoor environment. Regarding air pollution, I'm talking about more than automobile air pollution in our cities. I want you to consider more obscure, yet equally injurious, types of pollution that are found in rural and agricultural areas. Many pesticides, herbicides, and defoliants from farms enter the air when they're applied to crops, usually through crop dusting. According to the noted architect and environmental researcher Michael McDonough, in 2000 the number of people

Revitalize Your Hormones

Biological Age Assessment Quiz

Date _____

My chronological age is _____.

1. Based on what you check off, add and subtract the correspon-ding numbers from your chronological age.

2. Total up your biological age and address healing the issues that affect you.

General Health and Lifestyle

a. Your period is regular.

☐ yes   −1

☐ no   +1

b. The length of your last period was . . .

☐ 1 to 2 days   −1

☐ more than 5 days   +1

☐ 3 to 5 days   0

c. What are your current premenstrual   +1 each
syndrome symptoms?

☐ PMS 3 days to 2 weeks prior to menstruation

☐ premenstrual tension

☐ painful menses (cramping, etc.)

☐ excessive or prolonged menstruation

☐ painful/tender breasts

☐ too frequent menstruation

☐ acne, worse at menses

☐ depressed feelings before menstruation

☐ vaginal discharge

☐ scanty or missed menses

☐ depression

☐ hair loss

☐ insomnia

☐ abdominal bloating

☐ breast tenderness, swelling

☐ irritability, nervousness
☐ easy to anger, resentful
☐ feeling of being easily overwhelmed
☐ nausea and/or vomiting
☐ diarrhea or constipation
☐ headache
☐ food cravings, binge eating
☐ back pain
☐ feelings of faintness
☐ clumsiness
☐ forgetfulness
☐ weight gain—water

d. Dysplasia/fibrocystic syndrome   +2 each
☐ painful or tender lumps
☐ clear, gray, or yellow vaginal discharge
☐ vaginal bleeding after sex or between periods
☐ burning or itching on external genitalia
☐ urgent, painful urination
☐ lower abdominal or back pain
☐ heavy, watery, and bloody vaginal discharge
☐ heavy menstrual flow
☐ pelvic cramps
☐ thin, scant white vaginal discharge
☐ greenish yellow or offensive discharge
☐ cheesy white discharge
☐ breast lumps or swelling
☐ lumps that hurt just before period
☐ swelling under armpit
☐ change in breast size, shape
☐ white or slightly bloody vaginal discharge,
    one week prior to period
☐ current diagnosis of fibrocystic breast disease

e. Premenopause or menopause   +1 each
☐ difficulty sleeping

- [ ] hot flashes
- [ ] low libido
- [ ] exhaustion
- [ ] infertility
- [ ] frequent urination
- [ ] menstrual cycles greater than 32 days
- [ ] menstrual cycles less than 24 days
- [ ] absence of menstrual flow for six or more months
- [ ] occasional missed periods
- [ ] hair loss
- [ ] irregular menstrual cycle
- [ ] menses scanty or missed
- [ ] tubal ligation
- [ ] dry skin, hair
- [ ] lack of interest in sex
- [ ] mood swings, irritability
- [ ] depression, anxiety, nervousness
- [ ] craving for sweets, simple carbohydrates, binge eating
- [ ] headaches or dizziness
- [ ] painful intercourse
- [ ] spontaneous sweating
- [ ] shortness of breath and/or heart palpitations
- [ ] unpredictable vaginal bleeding
- [ ] vaginal dryness
- [ ] difficulty holding urine
- [ ] mental fogginess
- [ ] vaginal pain and/or itching
- [ ] thin, scant white vaginal discharge
- [ ] low back and/or hip pain
- [ ] breast tenderness, pain or tingling, prickling sensation
- [ ] easy bruising, loss of skin tone
- [ ] thinning armpit and pubic hair
- [ ] stopped menstruating
- [ ] breasts beginning to shrink, sag
- [ ] abnormal growth of hair above lip

General

a. Are you satisfied with your work, retirement, or school situation?

    ☐ happy with work, retirement, or school   −3

    ☐ unhappy with work, retirement, or school   +3

b. On a typical day, how many hours do you sleep?

    ☐ less than 6   +1

    ☐ 7 or 8 hours   −1

    ☐ 9 or more   +1

c. Are you overweight?

    ☐ weight is normal   −1

    ☐ 5 pounds   +2

    ☐ 10 to 20 pounds   +4

    ☐ more than 30 pounds   +5

d. Do you have extreme weight fluctuation?

    ☐ yes   +2

    ☐ no   0

e. How is the air quality you breathe?

    ☐ very clean   −1

    ☐ moderately clean   0

    ☐ polluted/smoggy   +2

f. Is your blood pressure . . . ?

    ☐ not sure   0

    ☐ high   +2

    ☐ low   −2

    ☐ normal   0

g.

    a. What is your cholesterol level?

        ☐ not sure   0

        ☐ high   +3

        ☐ low   −3

    b. What is your HDL (good) cholesterol level in mg/dl?

        ☐ not sure   0

        ☐ high   −3

        ☐ low   +3

h. Have you ever smoked cigarettes or cigars every day
   for 3 or *more months*?
   - ☐ yes   +2
   - ☐ no   −1

i. Do you currently smoke cigarettes, cigars, or a pipe?
   - ☐ yes
     - fewer than five cigarettes a day   +2
     - more than one pack a day   +5
   - ☐ no   −2

j. On a typical day, are you in an environment where people smoke?
   - ☐ yes   +2
   - ☐ no   0

k. Have you *ever* taken . . . ?
   - ☐ psychedelic drugs   +2
   - ☐ marijuana   +2

l. Have you ever had . . . ?   +3 each
   - ☐ breast cancer
   - ☐ ovarian cancer
   - ☐ other cancer
   - ☐ kidney disease
   - ☐ diabetes
   - ☐ cirrhosis
   - ☐ a stroke
   - ☐ a heart attack
   - ☐ asthma

m. Do you currently have . . . ?   +1 each
   - ☐ a virus
   - ☐ bacterial infection
   - ☐ vaginal yeast infection
   - ☐ fungal infection
   - ☐ parasites

n. Have you had any of the following surgeries?   +2 each
   - ☐ complete hysterectomy
   - ☐ tubal ligation

- ☐ partial hysterectomy
- ☐ pituitary/hypothalamus surgery
- ☐ thyroidectomy/partial or complete
- ☐ pineal surgery
- ☐ adrenal surgery
- ☐ kidney surgery
- ☐ gallbladder surgery
- ☐ liver surgery
- ☐ heart surgery
- ☐ colon surgery
- ☐ stomach surgery
- ☐ pancreas surgery
- ☐ spleen surgery
- ☐ brain surgery
- ☐ cancer/tumor surgery
- ☐ fibroid/cyst surgery

o. Family history

☐ cancer	+4
☐ heart disease	+3
☐ kidney disease	+2
☐ diabetes	+2

Nutrition

a. How often do you eat breakfast in a typical week?

☐ less than 1 time	+1
☐ 3 or more times	−1

b. Please check the following foods that you consume.

☐ whole grains	-5
☐ processed grains (white flour products)	+4
☐ junk food: pizza, burgers, fried chicken, potato chips, pretzels, soda, ice cream, donuts,	+5

    cakes, desserts, breakfast cereals coated with
        or containing sugar, and so on
☐   meat: beef, pork, chicken from the grocery   +4
        market (contains hormones and antibiotics)
☐   organic or hormone/antibiotic–free meats   +1
☐   fresh fish   −1
☐   3 to 5 servings of fresh vegetables per day   −4
☐   less than 2 servings of vegetables per day   +1
☐   dairy products: milk, butter, cream cheese,   +1
        cream, cheese
☐   eggs
        ☐   organic   −1
        ☐   not organic   +1
☐   daily processed soy products   +1
☐   organic fruits and vegetables   −4
☐   nonorganic fruits and vegetables   +1
☐   canola and other vegetable oils   +3
☐   olive oil   −3
☐   cooking fat and lard   +5

c. How often do you consume sugar, honey, maple
   syrup, fructose, or corn syrup?
   ☐   once a day   +1
   ☐   more than once a day   +2

d. Do you consume . . . ?
   ☐   natural sweetener: xylitol, mannitol,   −2
          sorbitol, stevia
   ☐   artificial sweetener: Equal, Saccharine,   +2
          Sweet'n Low, Splenda

e. Please enter how often you drink caffeinated
   beverages such as coffee, tea, and soda.
   ☐   one to three per week   −1
   ☐   one per day   +1
   ☐   two or more per day   +3

f. Please enter how many glasses of alcohol you drink
    (equivalent to one 12-ounce beer or one mixed drink).

    ☐ one to three per week   −1

    ☐ one per day   +1

    ☐ two or more per day   +2

g. Do you drink tap water?

    ☐ yes   +5

    ☐ no   −5

h. How much pure filtered water do you drink?

    ☐ none   +5

    ☐ less than six glasses per day   −2

    ☐ more than six glasses per day   −4

Physical Activities

a. How often do you do aerobic exercise
    (twenty-minute minimum)?

    ☐ never   +5

    ☐ twice per week   +1

    ☐ at least three times a week   −5

b. Please check the *nonaerobic health and fitness*   −2 each
    activities that you do at least three times per week

    ☐ yoga

    ☐ Pilates

    ☐ weight lifting

    ☐ tai chi or qi gong

    ☐ stretching

    ☐ other nonaerobic or noncardiovascular exercise

Stress, Social Support, and Spirituality

a. Do you meditate at least three times per week, have a spiritual
    practice, and/or attend church, synagogue, temple, mosque, or
    another place of meditation *at least* once a week?

    ☐ yes   −4

    ☐ no   +4

b. Please check if you have had a great deal of stress
   in the *last 24 months*.
   ☐ yes   +2
   ☐ no   –4

Medications

a. I am now taking the following medication . . .   +2 each
   ☐ birth control pills
   ☐ glucose-regulating drug
   ☐ SSRI
   ☐ thyroid medication
   ☐ Prozac, Celexa, Luvox, Paxil, or Effexor
   ☐ Remeron or Serzone
   ☐ Wellbutrin or Zyban
   ☐ Nardil, Parnate, or Marplan
   ☐ Elavil, Tofranil, or Sinequan
   ☐ Ritalin or Adderall

b. Please check how long you have used, in the past
   or currently, a *synthetic* hormone replacement.
   ☐ never   0
   ☐ 5 years or less   +3
   ☐ 6 to 11 years   +4
   ☐ 12 to 20 years   +5
   ☐ 21 or more years   +6

c. Please check how long you have used, in the past or currently,
   a *bio-identical compounded* hormone replacement.
   ☐ never   0
   ☐ 5 years or less   +1
   ☐ 6 to 11 years   +2
   ☐ 12 to 20 years   +3
   ☐ 21 or more years   +4

d. Please check how long you have used, in the past or currently, a
   natural progesterone or *wild yam cream* hormone replacement.
   ☐ never   0

☐	5 years or less	+1
☐	6 to 11 years	+2
☐	12 to 20 years	+3
☐	21 or more years	+4

e. Do you currently use the following?　　　　　　　　　−4 each
　　☐ herbal supplements
　　☐ vitamins and minerals
　　☐ homeopathy

poisoned by drifting pesticide in the United States had increased 20 percent from the previous year.

Many medical and scientific authorities consider the air quality in home and office environments critically important to our well-being. The U.S. Environmental Protection Agency (EPA) ranks indoor air pollution as one of the top five risks to public health. The fact is, indoor air pollution is an extra-strength version of outdoor air pollution.

New, tightly sealed buildings (where many of us work, live, or both) may keep toxin-laden vapors from chemically treated carpets, toxic building materials, plastic office furniture, cleaning products, and insecticides trapped inside, where they recirculate through the air and our bodies. When the polluting toxins are too tiny to be filtered by the lungs, they prevent oxygen from effectively entering the body and the bloodstream. Our upper respiratory system, lungs, heart, and circulatory and immune systems accumulate toxins; thus, their functioning is impaired. As a result, we may become more vulnerable to viruses, bacteria, and various diseases.

What Can Cause Allergies

It's estimated that approximately 60 percent of newly constructed homes contribute to our ill health. Toxicologists, allergists, and eco-conscious builders and designers describe this unfortunate situation as sick-building syndrome. You may wonder how sick-building syndrome relates to your endocrine system and hormones. The problem with "sick buildings" is that the toxins they release can tax your endocrine glands, thus contributing to endocrine breakdown and hormone imbalances. If you've recently moved into a new home or office and are experiencing persistent headaches, allergies, or other illnesses, it's entirely possible that toxins in the building are irritating your body.

We have all been exposed to various degrees of toxins on a daily basis for our entire lives. For instance, your digestive system almost continuously processes man-made carcinogens through the water you drink and the food you consume. It makes tragically perfect sense that nearly half of all cancers in the United States manifest in the digestive tract, with the colon the most cancer-stricken organ. High dietary fat and low fiber consumption are associated with slower movement through the gut, which allows food to ferment and putrefy, thus increasing the colon's exposure to potential cancer-causing substances.

Diet has a profound effect on colon cancer, as is evidenced by statistics showing that the rate of colon cancer in North Americans and Western Europeans is as much as ten times higher than in natives of Asia, Africa, and South America. The good news is that it's never too late to start detoxifying, feeling better, and safeguarding your health.

The Key to a Detoxified Body

Because it's in charge of ridding the body of cellular waste, the lymphatic system works at detoxifying your body twenty-four hours a day. As you may remember from high school biology, the lymphatic system is one of two principal circulating systems in the human body and encompasses capillaries, lymph fluid, lymph nodes, and ducts. The other major circulating system is, of course, the circulatory system, consisting of veins and arteries.

While the circulatory system delivers life-giving cellular nutrients and oxygen to special areas between the cells, the lymphatic system collects and processes excess fluid and particles from the tissues of the body, keeping the cells dry and efficient to ensure proper chemical and electrical balance and conductivity. Lymphatic fluid (also called lymph) contains white blood cells that fight infection and is therefore one of the strongest and most valuable players in your immune system.

Lymph nodes in the neck, the armpits, the abdomen, and the groin filter the lymph and attempt to destroy microorganisms and abnormal cells, which collect there. Cancer patients often have their lymph nodes removed to be examined for signs of malignant cells. Both the circulatory and the lymph system must work in tandem to maintain a healthy and dry cellular state.

When the lymph is dysfunctional, excess fluid and particles accumulate within the intercellular areas, resulting in inflammation. If the lymph stays immobilized and dysfunctional for extended periods, chronic inflammation occurs. Toxins from drugs, conventional or natural HRT, large protein molecules, processed food or water, and so on, begin to accumulate within the intercellular spaces and can provide a breeding ground for disease.

Detoxing the Lymph System

Along with regular aerobic exercise, one of the easiest ways to stimulate the lymphatic system is by dry brushing your body with a natural fiber brush, a loofah sponge, or a coarse natural fiber bath glove. Dry brushing also promotes blood circulation and oxygenation. Never use a nylon or synthetic fiber brush—the bristles are too sharp and may scrape your skin. Remember to always dry brush before you shower or bathe because you'll want to wash off the skin flakes that are produced by the brushing action.

Here's how to do it: begin with your feet and brush vigorously in circular motions. Brush away from your extremities and toward your heart. Continue brushing up your legs, then start on your hands and arms. Brush your entire back and abdomen area, shoulders, and neck. Brush around the breasts, under the armpits, and on the buttocks. Don't brush any sensitive, irritated, infected, or damaged areas of the skin and never dry brush facial skin. After brushing, take a shower or a bath. Doing this daily will help keep your lymphatic system and blood circulation in optimal shape.

Freshening Your Air

Indoor air purification units are excellent additions to any detoxification program. These cleaners imitate nature by duplicating its skillful filtration, dispersal, and ionization. Breathing clean, clear air brings more oxygen into your blood, which in turn helps your body to function at peak levels.

The square footage of a given room and the types of toxins you want to remove are key considerations when choosing an indoor air purification system. If you're lucky enough to live in a clean environment, you don't need this technology. However, if you live in a major metropolitan area, then, chances are, you'll benefit greatly from cleaning up the air supply in your home. If it's not within your budget to purify your entire home, focus on your bedroom. Since you spend a third of your life sleeping, just use an indoor air cleaner in the bedroom for fresh air while you rest.

Before you buy, remember that the most important things to look for are specific features, noise levels, and maintenance requirements/expense. Here's a rundown of some of the most effective types of indoor air purification units.

HEPA, or High Efficiency Particulate Arrestance Filters, are composed of intricate fiber networks. These trap at least 97 percent of all particles down to 0.3 microns in size, including asbestos, animal dander, bacteria, viruses, dust, pollen, mold, and tobacco smoke particles.

Carbon filters remove many pesticides, gaseous pollutants, volatile organic compounds, ozone, and various organic chemicals. They filter clean air by trapping pollutants in tiny recesses in the carbon.

Zeolites are natural minerals that neutralize odors and gaseous pollutants; these can be recharged by exposure to sunlight.

Electrostatic air cleaners include filters and precipitators. Both rely on a negative electric charge to attract and capture pollutants, including bacteria, molds, pollens, and toxic particulates like asbestos, animal dander, and tobacco smoke particles.

Ion exchange or ionization devices use negatively charged ions that attract positively charged pollutants into a filter that traps particles. Ion generators remove mainly smaller pollutants, such as tobacco smoke, smog particulates, and bacteria.

Corona discharge units function like lightning bolts, destroying toxins by using electronic plasma incineration. Use these to zap bacteria, dust, gases, molds, odors, viruses, and tobacco smoke particulates.

Detoxifying Your Water and Food

You can markedly reduce the amount of endocrine-disrupting organochlorines, arsenic, heavy metals, parasites, and other toxins you ingest by never drinking tap water or using ice cubes made from tap water. Instead, always drink purified or filtered water.

Please note that I do not refer to well-water here. While water from one well may be perfectly pure, well-water quality is influenced by several circumstances. These include the depth of the well and its proximity to sources of chemical pollutants, such as businesses, nuclear radiation storage facilities, nuclear plants, or underground storage tanks for gasoline. The latter frequently leak fuel additives and other toxins; the EPA reports that the fuel additive MTBE is found in virtually all drinking water around the country. As of this writing, EPA scientists are engaged in the absurd and alarming task of trying to establish what amount of MTBE is safe for human consumption.

I'm not trying to scare you; I simply want you to understand that just one small company can endanger an entire town's water supply or make it unfit for human consumption. If you'd like information on how to have your home water tested, go to the Web site www.epa. gov., where you'll find recommendations for water testing labs. The good news is that there are several effective purification/filtration options to choose from.

Various water filters are available today. Reverse osmosis is the best for removal of toxins, chemicals, bacteria, and viruses. There are under-the-counter, countertop, and whole-house models available. Alkaline water filters also offer an effective solution for purifying water. To further ensure that you always drink clean water, whenever you leave the house, carry purified bottled water with you so that you can maintain your detoxification regimen. Before buying bottled water, check the label first to see if it contains any chemical ingredients, sugar, fructose, sucralose, fluoride, arsenic, or heavy metals.

To purify shower water, use shower head attachments that filter out chlorine and other common chemicals. Bath faucet filters are somewhat effective in removing chlorine and other chemicals and will also spare you from inhaling chlorine and endocrine-disrupting organochlorines.

How to Detoxify Your Body

Use the notes you made on your symptoms when you reference the Five Element Body Clock on page 62. You'll know which organs need to be detoxified based on the times of the day or the night when your symptoms arise. To detoxify specific substances and organs, start with the detoxification diet and then move on to the homeopathic remedies in chapter 7.

One of the first and most important steps in detoxifying is doing a gallbladder/liver/kidney purification. This cleanses your liver, gallbladder, kidneys, and blood, while also boosting your immune system. It's vital to do this purification, because the liver conjugates hormones. A congested liver can cause hormonal problems such as hot flashes, an irregular menstrual cycle, premenopausal symptoms, headaches, and skin conditions.

Additional compelling reasons to do this flush include the fact that the gallbladder processes bile and fat. (These two substances can help to create gallstones and negatively affect hormone levels.) As you learned in chapter 2, the gallbladder also stores the neurotoxin and negative emotion called resentment. Over the last twenty years, I've helped patients, friends, and myself safely eliminate gallstones painlessly, while decongesting and detoxifying the liver. Gallbladder/liver flushes have been used in the holistic healing profession for at least two decades. Some of the old methods used by certain practitioners are too harsh for some people. The technique that I developed involves various wild-crafted herbs, minerals, fresh juices, and homeopathy.

The detoxification diet and the revitalization juice recipe found toward the end of this chapter will help you in this process.

Detoxification Guide

Detoxifying Medications and Conventional or Natural HRT

If you take (or have recently stopped using) any of the following medications, I recommend using the detoxification diet and homeopathy to detoxify your organs and support your health. I suggest that everyone, male and female alike, take a yearly Liver/Gallbladder/Kidney Cleanse (see the Resource Guide on how to order one) as a part of a three-week spring cleaning. Regarding homeopathic detoxification strategies for the following substances, please see chapter 7.

HRT/synthetic	any form of estrogen
HRT/"bio-identical"	any form of testosterone
"natural," OTC hormone	any form of estriol
replacement	Provera
any form of progesterone	Premarin

Estro-test	anti-inflammatory drugs
antibiotics	glucose-regulating drugs
antidepressants	thyroid medication
prednisone or cortisone	chemotherapy
heart medications	radiation
blood pressure medication	birth control pills

Any discussion of hormones and detoxification must also address the complicated, serious, and widely misunderstood topic of vaginal discharge. Caused by a constellation of factors, including toxins, drugs, oral contraceptives, yeast overgrowth, and STDs, vaginal discharge afflicts millions of women every day and can cause considerable discomfort. Knowing how to self-assess and self-treat vaginal discharge is a valuable part of your self-care and detoxification plan because it helps you to stay strong, healthy, and sexy.

Vaginal Discharge and Its Causes

Vaginitis with vaginal discharge is an extremely common problem, causing 10 million women each year to visit a physician's office for care. The three most common causes of vaginitis are bacterial, trichomonal, and fungal organisms. In as many as 75 percent of women with vaginitis, vulvovaginal candidiasis (yeast fungus) is the cause.

Bacterial vaginitis: May be caused by a host of organisms, including *Gardnerella vaginalis* (the most common), *Mobiluncus* species, *Mycoplasma hominis*, *Prevotella*, *Bacteroides*, and *Peptostreptococcus*. The two signs that help to confirm bacteria as the source of vaginitis are

1. the discharge is thin, homogeneous, and white and resembles skim milk adhering to the vaginal walls; and
2. the pH is above 4.5 (normal vaginal pH is 3.8–4.4); pH indicates the acid/alkaline balance in the body.

Trichomonal vaginitis: Causes a frothy, copious discharge that is yellowish or greenish and may have a fishy odor. In this condition, the vaginal pH exceeds 5–6. While many patients are asymptomatic, others report vaginal and vulvar discomfort, soreness, burning, and pain during sexual intercourse.

Candidal vaginitis: As many as 15 to 20 percent of females with vaginal yeast infections are asymptomatic. The reported symptoms of vaginal candidal infection are fairly characteristic and duplicative upon recurrence. They include vulvar and/or vaginal itching (which may be intense), burning soreness (especially when urinating), irritation, pain during intercourse, and the well-known curdlike discharge that adheres to the vaginal walls. Several noninfectious etiologies can produce similar symptoms.

Another clue in determining whether you have candidal vaginitis is the presence of a rash with a prominent border, similar to that in candida-infected diaper rash. The rash may spread outward from the vulvar area to involve the groin. The patient may also have satellite lesions outside the visible border. In worse cases, the patient may also experience chafing sores that scab over, the formation of pustules, and fissures of the labia.

Since nonprescription antifungals first became available more than a decade ago, millions of women have sought advice from pharmacists regarding self-care. Their number may well dwarf those who have made physician appointments. Today, many drugstore pharmacists are up to speed on homeopathy, and many cities have homeopathic pharmacies as well.

Situations That Mimic Vaginal Candidal Infection

Condition	Possible Causes
contact dermatitis	soaps, deodorants, underwear, detergents, spermicides, douche solutions, vaginal lubricants, perfumed cleansing wipes
irritant vulvitis	excessive use of minipads
vulvovaginitis	adverse reaction to vaginal antifungal product
change in vaginal mucus secretion	normal changes caused by ovulation
coitus-related vaginitis	allergy to partner's sperm

Species of Candida

Candida albicans is able to adhere to vaginal epithelium more readily than other Candida species are, which is probably why it causes about 80 percent of yeast infections. Other less common causes are *C. glabrata*, *C. parapsilosis*, *C. guilliermondii*, and *C. tropicalis*.

For two hundred years, homeopathy has been used to remedy all of the previously mentioned conditions. (A homeopathic remedy is available, including vaginal suppositories, for all of these conditions; see chapter 7.) You'll find information on where to obtain remedies in the Resource Guide.

Immune Health and Candidal Infections

A compromised immune system can also induce candidal infection. Using systemic corticosteroids and having AIDS are both associated with infection. Diabetes, glucosuria, lupus, thyroid dysfunction, and obesity are thought to be predisposing factors as well.

Much research has proved that antibiotic use can increase candida vaginitis risk through alteration of the intravaginal flora. Apparently, antibiotics upset the reciprocal balance between normal vaginal organisms through the eradication of bacteria. Research and my own clinical experience indicate that some of the antibiotics that can foster candidal infection include ampicillin, tetracycline, clindamycin, and the cephalosporins. (Many gynecology and internal medicine textbooks report the same connection.)

Easy Preventive Strategies

On the more everyday front, certain types of clothing may predispose people to developing candida. For example, you should avoid wearing tight-fitting clothes and synthetic underwear, which can promote candida growth. I know this is the last thing that some women want to hear, but frequent coitus and the use of intrauterine devices may also contribute to infections. Women should rule out bathing in hot tubs or Jacuzzis too often, and they should also avoid any situation in which the outer vaginal area is exposed to prolonged moisture, such as wearing a wet bathing suit throughout a long summer day at a pool or a water park. The chemically treated water in hot tubs and overly chlorinated swimming pool water may also cause candida through irritation of delicate vulvar/vaginal tissues.

Some research indicates that 80 percent of women do not recognize the signs of bacterial vaginitis (BV), the most common and potentially serious form of vaginal infection. They may confuse the signs of BV for a yeast infection and thus self-treat inappropriately with OTC drugs that are meant to eradicate candidal infection. If you self-treat using the correct homeopathic remedy or suppository, however, the results can be swift and permanent.

Treatment Considerations

Patients with candidal vaginitis should take special care of the vulvar region. They should avoid the use of harsh soap and perfumes and should keep the vulvar area dry to discourage overgrowth. Vulvar itching may be controlled by careful application of a topical vaginal antifungal. Nonprescription hydrocortisone may enhance the antifungal's effectiveness.

The problem with using any drug, according to homeopathic or European naturopathic training, is that drugs suppress the condition, rather than heal it. For example, this is why some people who take antibiotics for bronchitis experience recurrent infections throughout the year. On the other hand, homeopathic products are effective and will actually relieve the burning, discharge, and itching of vaginal yeast infections, and they are approved by the FDA. You'll learn more about these in chapter 7.

Vaginal Fungal (Yeast) Infections

Vaginal fungal infections are a common and troubling nuisance for many women. Whereas you must follow specific instructions and be aware of precautions regarding side effects before you attempt self-treatment with OTC drugs, homeopathy has no side effects. You should feel better within three to ten days of homeopathic treatment.

The point I want to reiterate about this self-assessment and the homeopathic approach is that it cures. Drugs merely suppress symptoms and keep them at bay until we experience more stress and then the symptoms return again.

What to Do If the Condition Returns

Vaginal fungal infections often return if you use OTC or prescription drugs. Look for a different diagnosis and see a holistic health provider to discover whether you are pregnant or have AIDS or diabetes. Also, read the information on inherited toxins in this chapter to gain insight into how to care for your condition.

Understanding Types of Toxins

Acquired Toxins

When I studied homeopathy in Germany with physicists and biophysicists, I learned about toxins found in the environment, our food, prescription drugs, and so on, and how these may affect the human body. (They are called acquired toxins.) I also learned how to locate and eliminate toxins in my patients by using homeopathic remedies, which are derived from plants, minerals, and other substances. Now I'd like to discuss some of the various types of toxins and how to treat them, according to the European naturopathic and homeopathic medical models. (Homeopathic remedies for detoxifying the body of acquired and inherited toxins are discussed in detail in chapter 7.)

Inherited Toxins

Advanced studies in homeopathic and bioenergetic medicine reveal that certain toxins are passed on through our genes from generation to generation. They can lie dormant for years before surfacing as an illness. Inherited toxins are known to be a taint in the cells that can trigger common health conditions such as asthma, psoriasis, pulmonary problems, mental illness, dysbiosis, candida, and arthritis, just to name a few. All of the remedies for the following inherited toxins can be found in chapter 7.

Here's an overview of inherited toxins:

Toxoplasmosis: This is a parasite whose host is the house cat. Infection often occurs from the consumption or the handling of meat or from contact with cat feces. Pregnant women should avoid contact with cats and should never empty litter pans. Symptoms may resemble mononucleosis, with chills, fever, headache, and general aches.

Salmonella: This bacteria enters the body through contaminated food and water. Symptoms include chronic gastroenteritis, food poisoning, gastrointestinal ulceration, Crohn's disease, and gastric headaches.

Influenzinum: This refers to all strains of influenza. Practically any tissue in the body can harbor these tenacious viruses. A full range of flu-like symptoms can plague people with this.

Medorrhinum: Also known as gonorrhea. Symptoms may include chronic ovarian ailments, uterine fibroids, cysts, and other uterine and ovarian growths or disease; also, any acute carcinomas or cancers.

Syphillinum: Also known as syphilis. People who have this inherited toxin may experience constant headaches, memory impairment, asthma, sciatica, frequent abscesses, hair loss, and swollen legs. Emotional symptoms can be serious, manifesting as fearing the night, fearing that one is going insane, or fearing imminent paralysis.

Tuberculinum: Also known as tuberculosis and referred to as TB. Symptoms include a propensity to catch colds, arthritis, acute rheumatism, nervous weakness, tonsillitis, exhaustion, epilepsy, and rapid emaciation.

Naturopathic theory posits that an inherited toxin can morph into an illness that may not resemble the exact symptoms associated with the specific toxin. For example, tuberculosis can morph into asthma or pneumonia, and the symptoms of these two illnesses are, for the most part, different from those of TB. The following case history highlights how inherited toxins can profoundly affect health.

Joanna visited me for detoxification and nutritional balancing after her lungs collapsed, causing her to be hospitalized for a week. She explained that the diagnosis was asthma, and that she had experienced all of the normal asthmatic symptoms since childhood. At the time, Joanna was taking five prescription medications, including the steroid drug Prednisone, and was using an inhaler and oxygen.

After I took a lengthy medical history, during which I inquired whether anyone in her family had any of the inherited toxins described previously, she replied no. I performed NeuroPhysical Reprogramming, or NPR, a technique that I developed. (It's a program approved by the California Bureau of Private Post-Secondary and Vocational Education that treats physical, mental, and emotional conditions. NPR is detailed in chapter 6, which covers emotional self-management. There I outline a crucial healing step from the

NPR process that you can learn quickly and start to practice immediately.)

To my surprise, I discovered that her body tested for tuberculosis, bronchitis, and pneumonia. I again asked if anyone in her family had tested positive for TB, and she again replied no.

The next day, after Joanna questioned her parents, her father answered that he had tested positive for TB many years ago. (I've learned that my being a persistent detective benefits my patients greatly.) I tested Joanna for the correct homeopathic TB remedy and potency, and after she took it for five days, her asthma symptoms began to lessen. Joanna felt her energy shift, and she started walking for exercise, which she hadn't done in a year or more.

Because Joanna had been adjusting her medications over the years, she started to reduce her drug dosages slowly and safely, until she cut them out, one by one. Besides the homeopathic remedies that Joanna took, she also used the detox diet in this chapter, drinking revitalization juice and wheat grass juice, along with using the Food Pyramid on page 102. I also recommended a small amount of nutritional supplements, such as rutin, bioflavonoids, buffered vitamin C, a women's multivitamin made from whole foods, enzymes to help control inflammation, and an immunity-stimulating mushroom formula to help take the place of her medications. Her asthma is now effectively under control.

I'm not suggesting that you stop taking your medications without a holistic medical provider's assistance. I reported this case history to demonstrate that it is possible to cure asthma, and many other diseases, for that matter, with natural remedies. Unfortunately, most consumers never even hear the specifics of natural healing or strategies for detoxifying.

Skin Care Clean-Up

We all understand the meaning of the expression "you are what you eat." In the case of skin care products, you are what you wear, for whatever you apply to your skin ends up in your bloodstream and inside your body. For this reason, I advise off-loading any cleansers, toners, scrubs, astringents, makeup removers, or moisturizers that contain animal products or petroleum derivatives, like the chemical paraben twins, methyl and poly. Furthermore, get rid of anything that contains chemicals you can't pronounce. In their place, use organic skin care products that are based on botanical or marine extracts. You'll find a list of organic skin care companies in the Resource Guide.

Makeup, Skin, and Hair Care Detox

Any worthwhile detoxification plan must include lightening the toxic load that your body ironically acquires through self-care and beautification. Conventional hair dyes, nail polishes, and other color cosmetics either contain known toxins and carcinogens or are petrochemically based. Many fabulous alternatives are available, though—namely, nontoxic, organic plant and/or mineral-based hair dyes and color cosmetics. You can find these in health food stores and day spas, on the Internet, and in beauty supply shops.

Skin and hair care preparations made from organic plants are soothing, beautifying, and toxin-free. Realize that whenever you beautify yourself with these organic products, you reap multiple health and beauty benefits while you support a cleaner environment. Talk about makeup that matters—and good hair days! The farmers who grow organic plants that are used for body and hair care blends never use toxic pesticides, herbicides, or chemical fertilizers. Organic farmers are, in essence, detoxifying our water, soil, and air. They are benefiting all living beings and deserve to be supported by consumers.

Besides being hypoallergenic, mineral color cosmetics are vibrant and cost-effective. Pure mineral color cosmetics nourish and protect the skin with anti-inflammatory properties and natural sunscreen. (Many mineral powder cosmetics contain SPF 15 or higher, without the harsh chemicals found in many conventional sunscreens.)

Three-Month Endocrine-Rebuilding Diet

The best time to embrace health is now, so start this diet as soon as you can. You need not make any changes to jump right into this healing diet, except for taking a trip to the health food store to stock up on organic foods. *Hint:* The recipes in part 3 make it easy, fast, and fun for you to prepare delicious, hormone-balancing foods at every meal, even if you brown bag it for your lunch. I also recommend that you keep a diet diary. Jot down a few sentences about how your body feels and what your energy level is each day.

For the last thirty years, I've used the endocrine-rebuilding diet as my basic tool and my passport for staying healthy, vital, and sexy. In opposition to high-protein diet fads, my studies in naturopathic and homeopathic healing indicate that animal protein is not the most healthful food for the body. Because I prefer to consume my protein through organic beans, brown rice, tempeh, wild fish, and homemade seed and nut milks, my diet contains extremely small amounts of animal protein.

My patients who had critical hormone imbalances all responded beautifully to the endocrine-rebuilding diet. The amount of live foods and the absence of animal protein in this eating plan make it far easier for the body to assimilate essential nutrients; therefore, the body is provided with more nourishment.

This immensely effective diet helps to balance metabolism while deep cleansing the body, restoring immune function, and revitalizing the endocrine system. I have used this plan and prescribed it to patients for the last two decades. It involves eating three meals daily and two raw vegetable or seed snacks.

This diet is for detoxification purposes and to assist with rebuilding the endocrine system. It is not meant to diagnose or cure disease. As individual needs may vary, please consult with your holistic health-care provider. Use the optimum health breakfast and deep cleansing recommendations for the first month. Eat frequently. The second and third months, add some more oils, seeds, legumes, and other proteins, as listed in the following paragraphs.

This diet plan consists of approximately 70 percent raw foods. Because raw foods contain all of their enzymes, vitamins, and minerals, they are nutritionally superior to cooked foods, which lose nutrient value during heating. To promote optimum health and digestion, this diet also incorporates certain rules of food combining, such as never combining eggs or any other type of protein with carbohydrates, such as bread or fruit.

Buy everything organic, if possible, including poultry and fish. (This means avoiding farmed salmon and other fish.) You can order organic foods over the Internet if they're unavailable in your area. If you are estrogen-dominant, avoid soy because it could make your estrogen levels higher. I have patients who are so soy-obsessed that they eat massive amounts of soy each day in the form of soy milk, soy nuts, soy cheese, soy dessert, soy protein drinks, soybeans, and tofu. While they're very well-meaning, soy food fanatics are making dietary mistakes.

Rather than go overboard on processed soy foods, it's far more healthful to eat whole steamed soybeans, called edamame. These beans are healthful to eat in moderate amounts and will not adversely affect estrogen levels or inhibit thyroid function. Sprouted grains may be tolerable, even with gluten and wheat intolerance. (People who want, or need, to avoid gluten should bear in mind that the only two gluten-free grains are rice and corn.) For more information on gluten tolerance and other food allergens, I recommend that you visit www.csaceliacs.org, the medically authoritative yet extremely helpful Web site of the Celiac Sprue Association.

Please note that the following foods include individual meal suggestions.

Should you desire to do a deep cleanse, you must abstain from eating animal protein for thirty days and instead combine legumes and grains. A daily sauna, a colonic, and/or an enema can also be very helpful in the detoxification process. So can drinking 2 ounces of wheat grass juice five days a week. Before I outline the diet, here's an important warning for women who have been diagnosed as estrogen-dominant. Avoid the following substances and herbs: soy, licorice, red clover, thyme, turmeric, hops, and verbena. They are estradiol-binding, which means that they increase the amount of estrogen in your system.

Breakfast

Raw organic fruit: watermelon and other melons (but not for patients with blood sugar problems); berries

Organic muesli

Organic raw seeds

Organic sprouted flourless bread or manna bread

Organic macadamia nut or almond smoothie

Original flavor almond milk (find one with a low sugar gram content)

Optimum Health Breakfast Choices

Fresh vegetable juice (but no carrots or beets for patients with blood sugar problems)

Sesame and pumpkin seed smoothie (for people who need more protein and have been cleansing for two weeks)

Note: Seeds and nuts must be soaked overnight to break down enzyme inhibitors so that they're easier to digest. Blend them on the highest setting and add purified water to taste. Make enough for one 8-ounce glass.

Lunch and Dinner

Vegetables: raw salads with avocado, tomatoes, celery, spinach, string beans, cucumber, zucchini, cilantro, onions, and anise

Animal protein: As mentioned earlier, this is not recommended if you're doing a deep cleanse.

Choose one of the following per lunch: organic poultry, or a very small portion of grains and vegetables.

Raw organic cheese (once weekly)

Deep-sea wild fish, such as salmon

Beans or lentils (legumes) and brown rice combined make a protein.

Grains (organic whole grains): Corn and brown rice are best because they are gluten-free.

Raw corn is delicious and sweet. Ancient grains such as spelt, quinoa, and amaranth are excellent, except they do contain small amounts of gluten.

Oils:

One tablespoon of a combination of organic flaxseeds (ground), borage oil, and evening primrose oil daily.

Use organic olive oil in all cooking and on salads.

Use organic raw butter once or twice per week if desired.

Do not fry or overheat food, as it destroys enzymes. You may warm foods, but never fry or overheat oil.

Note: If you are deep cleansing, the only appropriate oils to consume are organic olive oil or flaxseed oil. Oil should never be
heated. It is used in salads to balance hormones.

Beverages

Drink eight 8-ounce glasses of alkaline water daily. You can find
this in health food stores.

You may also drink noncarbonated vegetable juices and herbal
teas, including chaste tree tea, which helps to balance hormones.

The more pure alkaline water you drink, the more effective the
detoxification.

Snacks

If you must eat something sweet, wheat- and gluten-free vegan
cookies are the best options.

Organic fresh or dehydrated fruit

Organic raw almonds, organic macadamia nuts, pumpkin or
sesame seeds (soak nuts overnight)

Macrobiotic hard candy, wheat- and yeast-free crackers, popcorn
(no butter)

Organic raw sunflower seeds, sesame seeds, and hulled pumpkin
seeds are healthful snacks.

Stevia and/or brown rice syrup should replace *all* sugars.

Deep Cleanse

Wheat grass juice is used for detoxification and can be drunk on a
regular basis. This is one of the most vital foods on the planet, brim-
ming with life-giving vitamins, amino acids, and minerals. Doctors
recommend drinking 2 to 4 ounces of wheat grass daily, one hour
between eating any food.

Wheat grass juice must be consumed immediately after juicing it.
You can buy this at juice and smoothie shops and health food stores.
The most economical way to work wheat grass juice into your diet is
to purchase flats of wheat grass from the health food store, along
with a wheat grass juicer, and juice it yourself.

Foods to Avoid during Deep Cleansing

The foods in the following list should never be eaten during a deep cleanse or consumed on a regular basis. This is because they exert various detrimental effects on the body, plus trigger known allergies, which can sometimes contribute to endocrine breakdown. Some common examples that may affect your health include caffeine, which exhausts and dehydrates the adrenal glands, and alcohol, which, depending on the type and the strength, negatively affects the pancreas, the adrenal glands, and the liver. (In small amounts, organic wine and sake may be easier on your body than conventional alcohol is.)

As mentioned previously, fried foods and trans fats age the body and should be avoided.

yeast	cakes
chocolate	candy
alcohol	meat and poultry that is not
sodas	organically raised
refined sugars	MSG
artificial sweetener	soy and tofu
gluten	all dairy
food preservatives	fried foods
caffeine	shellfish

Revitalizing Juice Recipe

Drink at least 8 ounces daily for the first month, then continue four times per week thereafter. Juice the following *organic* produce items into an 8-ounce glass. My patients report that drinking 16 ounces per day does wonders for their energy, elimination, moods, and skin.

1 medium-sized carrot

1 medium-sized beet

dandelion greens (These are bitter, so add them to taste. The more you add, the deeper the cleanse for your liver and gallbladder.)

collard greens

kale

cucumber

parsley

celery

a little fresh ginger root, to taste

½ apple (If you have been diagnosed with diabetes or have blood
sugar problems, eliminate the apple, carrot, and beet.)

After following the endocrine-rebuilding diet for three months,
your endocrine function will become more efficient so that it can
start producing and balancing hormones in appropriate amounts.
In the next chapter, you'll learn about nutritional support strategies
for various endocrine-related health conditions, as well as other
illnesses.

What to Do after Three Months on the Diet

You have many choices now. You can continue to feel great by
using this diet and the hormone-balancing recipes for the rest of your
life. Or, you can use the diet as a healing tool, modifying it now and
then by adding occasional treats. When the diet is over, look back to
see how you felt four months ago. Then assess the situation to determine whether you need to continue on the diet for three more
months.

You can also retake the biological age assessment and the other
self-assessments in this book to see how much younger and sexier
you've become. Let your results and your libido be your guide. I
always say, if it isn't broken, never change a thing.

Step 3 Action Plan

1. Take the biological age assessment to determine the nature of your
   health.
2. Detoxify your body and strengthen your endocrine system by cutting out sugar, caffeine, alcohol, cigarettes, chemically preserved
   foods, any form of HRT, and, if possible, any prescription drugs
   you are taking.

3. Do a Liver/Gallbladder/Kidney Cleanse (see the Resource Guide, to order a kit for this).
4. Detoxify the air and the water in your house by purchasing the appropriate filters.
5. Carefully study the symptoms of inherited toxins to determine whether you have any of them. Talk to family members to establish whether these symptoms were experienced by your parents or grandparents.
6. Mark the start date to begin your detoxification diet on your calendar.
7. Go to the health food store for the items you need. Here's a shopping list:

    organic green, yellow, red, and white vegetables

    organic brown rice (After trying brown rice, you may also try spelt, kamut, teff, and quinoa.)

    stainless steel steamer for vegetables

    organic salad dressing with olive oil and *no* sugar or honey

    organic tomato sauce without sugar or honey

    organic condiments such as mustard, eggless safflower mayonnaise, and ketchup, all without sugar

    Celtic sea salt, organic black pepper

    organic balsamic vinegar

    organic olive oil

    organic seasonings, such as whole fresh garlic, onions, red curry powder, cumin, basil, and cayenne pepper

    pure reverse osmosis water or alkaline water such as Essentia

    stainless steel or glass CorningWare cookware

    organic poultry and wild deep-sea fish

    organic rice milk

    organic fruit: watermelon for cleansing in the morning, if you don't have a blood sugar problem; fresh or frozen berries; young whole coconut (Get help with opening this to drink the clear, delicious juice that some islanders call "coconut water"— not to be confused with coconut milk, which is made by grating or pulverizing the coconut meat, then squeezing out the creamy white liquid.) Or, scrape out the white coconut meat to eat or put in a smoothie.

organic teas without caffeine

organic coffee substitute, such as Teeccino

Get a stove, use a convection oven, and throw away your microwave oven.

8. Drink at least 8 ounces of revitalization juice each day.

9. Drink at least 2 ounces of wheat grass juice five days a week.

Step 4

Food, Glorious Food: Hormone-Revitalizing Diet and Nutrition

Julia had taken birth control pills for more than fifteen years and now wanted to become pregnant. She had tried for just over a year without any success before she came to me.

Like many women whom I help, Julia had dieted consistently for quite a few years and had followed various regimens at different times. One that she used consistently was a low-fat, high-carbohydrate diet. My patients with hormone problems have often tried multiple diets and, as a result, are deficient in many essential nutrients.

I gave Julia a hormone-balancing diet tailored especially for her. The most important foods I added were those rich in omega-3 essential fatty acids. These good fats are essential for building hormones. Many patients who swear to me that they eat healthfully turn out to be deficient in these.

Julia followed my Seven-Step Program, using the Food Pyramid Chart to guide her, and after six months she became pregnant. Each aspect of the program was a crucial contribution to her improvement. She felt much more energetic and clear-headed after adhering to a nutritious diet that was designed to balance her hormones, and it gave her the nourishment necessary to coproduce and grow a new life.

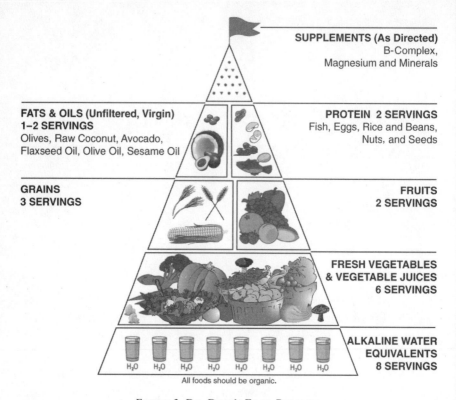

FATS & OILS (Unfiltered, Virgin)
1-2 SERVINGS
Olives, Raw Coconut, Avocado,
Flaxseed Oil, Olive Oil, Sesame Oil

SUPPLEMENTS (As Directed)
B-Complex,
Magnesium and Minerals

PROTEIN 2 SERVINGS
Fish, Eggs, Rice and Beans,
Nuts, and Seeds

GRAINS
3 SERVINGS

FRUITS
2 SERVINGS

FRESH VEGETABLES
& VEGETABLE JUICES
6 SERVINGS

ALKALINE WATER
EQUIVALENTS
8 SERVINGS

All foods should be organic.

FIGURE 3: DR. DALE'S FOOD PYRAMID

In the last chapter, you learned that what you eat can decrease your biological age, making your body younger than your chronological age. In this chapter, you'll learn which specific foods and supplements will help you balance and build your hormones. My Food Pyramid Chart helps you plan the portions of each type of food to eat on a daily basis. It's quite simple: the largest portion at the bottom of the chart consists of drinking water. As you move up the chart, you'll see vegetables and so on.

As Julia discovered, eating well is an enjoyable, simple, and practical way to revitalize hormones naturally. Balanced nutrition supports the endocrine glands that produce your hormones, as well as all your other organs and body systems. Eating good, fresh, unprocessed food can also help you look your best and will make you feel like a teenager, energized and sexy.

Eating well is a matter of urgent concern to me. According to the American Obesity Association (AOA), the prevalence of obesity among adults rose 60 percent nationally since 1991. Scientists know that this enormous increase in such a brief period of time cannot be blamed solely on genetic factors. Much compelling research indicates that the rise in obesity is generated by our behavior, such as our eating habits, diet, exercise levels, and computer use.

While chapter 3 discussed toxins in foods, I want to stress here that the average American diet contains many *toxic foods*, such as sodas, food coloring, sugar substitutes made from synthetic chemicals, and trans-fatty acids from fried foods. All of these foods make your organs and body systems age faster than normal healthful organic foods do and thus increase your biological age, while upsetting your hormone balance. Believe me, there's a better way to eat.

There are many delicious foods that will help you bring your hormones into comfortable, efficient balance, while providing the nutrients for you to enjoy vibrant health. This chapter will show you how to achieve hormone balance and how to eat to maintain your optimum weight. I'll tell you which foods to eliminate from your refrigerator and cupboards and how to stock your pantry. But first, I'll say a few words about food toxicity, which should help you gauge whether your eating habits are off balance.

Food Toxicity

Food toxicity results from not eating properly or from following protein-heavy designer diets. If you eat too much of one type of food, like animal protein, for too long, it can become a toxin to your body. This rule underlies Chinese Five Element Medical Theory, as well as naturopathic healing. Your body gets out of balance by consuming too much of one substance over long periods of time. (Vegetables are the exception. You can safely eat large amounts of organically grown vegetables for the rest of your life, and they will only contribute to your good health.)

My patients who've tried high-protein celebrity diets feel much better when they stop eating animal protein and ignore those advertisements urging them to try the other white meat! For protein, I recommend eating whole-grain brown rice or wild rice combined with various beans, lentils, or tempeh (a delicious fermented soybean product that's available in health food stores). Another good protein source is organic hemp or whey protein powder, which you can mix into smoothie drinks.

The recommended daily allowance (RDA) of protein may be inappropriate for your body's needs, just as the protein recommendations in fad diets may be wrong for you. You're not a statistic, you're a human being with emotions, and you are biochemically unique! Your protein and carbohydrate needs will vary according to your stress levels (which change daily, according to unexpected events), exercise, and biological age. Furthermore, body size can dictate protein needs: a female pro basketball player and a naturally petite woman will have dramatically different protein requirements.

Comfort foods, such as pastries, potatoes, bread, pasta, and pizzas, are a major source of carbohydrates. My case histories indicate that even these beloved carbs can become toxins to the body, as they can cause neurotransmitter imbalances that trigger hormone imbalances.

No discussion of food toxicity is complete without mentioning eating disorders, which are more prevalent among women than among men and often start to manifest in the teenage years. Eating disorders inevitably create endocrine and neurotransmitter imbalances, not to mention the havoc they wreak on one's mood and state of mind. Eating disorders sabotage the body's attempts to digest food and obtain the nutrients it needs to make hormones and other essential substances in appropriate amounts. Any eating disorder can be cured through awareness tools that help release old belief systems and identify the anchor health condition. Support groups may be helpful to discuss your feelings; however, this does not take the place of effective tools to access and release the cause of the disorder. Homeopathy is a very effective tool for this purpose.

Now is the time to survey the foundations of a hormone-revitalizing diet, and the most healthful way to eat for you, your hormones, the environment, and future generations.

Acid/Alkaline Balance and Our Health

Understanding how the acid/alkaline balance of the food we eat affects our health is key to maintaining a healthy body and balanced hormones. Studies show that the standard American diet includes a mere 20 to 30 percent alkaline food, whereas we should be eating at least 70 to 80 percent alkaline and 20 to 30 percent acid food.

Good health requires eating foods that replenish our body's alkalinity on a daily basis. A food is considered alkaline if it contains organic minerals and is deemed acid if the residue that remains after the food is digested, processed, and metabolized contains inorganic acid. Whether a food is acid or alkaline depends on its ash value. Ash value refers to the type of residue that remains after the food is metabolized, digested, and processed. This residue, called ash, contains certain chemical and metallic substances. If the ash residue is acid, the body must neutralize this to prevent the blood from becoming too acidic. The acid must be neutralized by something that's alkaline, hence the importance of eating alkaline foods.

A healthful diet will create adequate alkalinity to keep you vital and strong. In contrast, an unhealthful diet that contains mostly acid-forming foods will cause your body to extract alkalinity from the cells, in order to neutralize the acid. Moreover, this leaching of alkalinity from the cells creates acidity and leaves you vulnerable to disease.

An acid and alkaline balance must be maintained for us to experience consistent good health. If we consume too many acid-forming foods, the cellular pH of our bodies becomes too acid. If this condition persists for too long, we may feel out of sorts or ill. Since the body doesn't manufacture organic minerals, we must regularly consume alkaline foods to avoid becoming too acidic.

The following acid/alkaline scale reveals the variation between alkaline and acid pH.

Symptoms of an Acid Condition

Don't be concerned if you have any of the following symptoms, which are associated with an acid condition. This chapter contains a wealth of suggestions to help you resolve the problem.

Acid Symptoms

insomnia	migraine headaches
water retention	alternating constipation and
rheumatoid arthritis	diarrhea

frequent colds or flus   bumps on the tongue

difficulty swallowing   stomach ulcers

burning in the mouth   acid reflux

The acid/alkaline scale shown here reveals variations between alkaline and acid pH. The pH is a measure of how acid or how alkaline a substance is. The pH scale, ranging from 1 to 14, determines a substance's level of acidity or alkalinity.

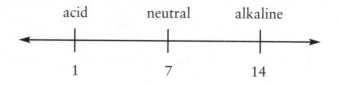

Alkaline and Acid Foods

Most high-protein foods (such as meat, fish, poultry, and eggs) and nearly all carbohydrates (including grains, breads, and pastas) and fats are acid forming. On the other hand, most fruits and vegetables are alkaline forming. Citrus fruits, such as oranges and grapefruit, contain organic acids and have an acidic taste, but they're not acid forming. When citrus fruits are metabolized, they create an alkaline residue.

It's helpful to remember that all processed and fried foods are acid. Because coffee is acid forming, your daily cup of coffee just might eliminate any alkalinity that you've developed over the day. I hate to be the bearer of bad news, but soft drinks, spirits, and wine are even more acid-producing. The good news is that we will look at examples of how to balance acid and alkaline foods to build a healthy and sexy body.

You will combine your foods with one simple rule in mind: 50 percent of your meal will include at least two varieties of raw or steamed vegetables. Choose one green vegetable (for its chlorophyll and mineral content) and any other vegetable. For breakfast, make a green drink (see the revitalizing juice recipe in chapter 3) or, if you have no blood sugar problems, eat organic berries or watermelon. If you have a juicer, juice a variety of vegetables and drink to your health.

In the hierarchy of food alkalinity, raw vegetables and fruit are the most alkaline, steamed vegetables are next, and boiled foods are the least alkaline and most acid. To help you start to balance your diet, here's a list of alkaline-forming and acid-forming foods.

Alkaline-Forming Foods

almonds	grapes
apricots	honey
avocados	lemons
blackstrap molasses	lima beans
brazil nuts	maple syrup
buckwheat	melons
chestnuts	millet
coconuts (fresh)	oranges
corn	raisins
dates	soy/tempeh
figs	vegetables
grapefruit	wheat grass

Acid-Forming Foods

alcohol	fruit (canned/glazed)
asparagus	fruit (dried and sulfured)
beans	grains (most)
brussels sprouts	ice cream
butter	legumes
catsup	lentils
cheeses	meat
chickpeas	milk
cocoa	mustard
coconuts (dried)	noodles
coffee	nuts (most)
cornstarch	oatmeal
eggs	olives
fish	pasta
flour products	pepper

poultry   soft drinks
sauerkraut   sugar
seeds   tea
shellfish

What's an Acid pH?

An acid pH, or "acidosis," describes an imbalanced acidic state, which affects all of our body fluids. The pH of our body's various fluids, such as blood, urine, and saliva, strongly influences all cellular functions. If the pH swings too far to the acid side, cells become poisoned in their own toxic acidic wastes, and they die.

A good way to understand acid/alkaline balance is to review our temperature, which is normally balanced at 98.6 degrees Fahrenheit. If our temperature becomes several degrees out of balance, we can become very ill. Maintaining our pH balance is far more critical, however, because the *slightest* imbalance can cause serious illness and disease.

The body regulates itself the best it can, doing whatever is necessary to maintain pH balance. It performs this task by continually stealing acid-neutralizing minerals (such as calcium) from the bones in an attempt to maintain health. This explains why elderly people who have a meat-heavy diet often develop osteoporosis, after a lifetime of consuming acid-producing foods. Remember, fresh fruits and vegetables are alkaline producing and help your body maintain a healthy pH balance.

Why You Should Know about Your pH

It's a well-known medical fact that a consistent acid pH is dangerous. Just think about "acid rain" and how it destroys the natural environment, killing plants and trees, poisoning the life in lakes and rivers. An acid pH, however, is even more dangerous than acid rain, because it continuously corrodes all body tissue. An acid pH can interrupt all cellular activities and functions, from the beating of your heart to the functioning of your brain. Therefore, I'm providing some guidelines for giving yourself a pH checkup.

How Do I Know Whether I Have an Acid pH?

You may test your pH level in the privacy of your own home. A good rule is to test your urine upon waking in the morning or at least one hour after eating, according to the method detailed in the next section. When urinary pH is *continuously* between 7.0 and 7.5, you're functioning in a healthy range. If urine tests less than 6.8 pH, you are too acid, and readings over 7.5 pH mean you are too alkaline. As you can see from the pH scale on page 106, a pH below 7.0 is acid, while anything with a pH above 7.0 is alkaline.

Now that you understand the importance of maintaining a balanced alkaline and acid pH and how foods affect your pH, you can test your pH by using the following method.

Acid and Alkaline Self-Test

This empowering self-test will help you monitor your progress by assessing whether your body fluids are either too acidic or too alkaline. This system of checks and balances can alert you if you have the conditions known as acidosis or alkalosis.

The best plan is to test yourself as soon as possible to get a good baseline pH reading, and then again a couple of weeks after starting your hormone revitalization diet, which is detailed later in this chapter.

To do the test, you'll need to purchase nitrazine (test strips) paper from any drugstore. To achieve the most accurate reading, perform this test before eating or at least one hour after eating. The paper comes with simple instructions that help you interpret your acid and alkaline levels. Hold the paper under the urine stream and follow the instructions. Write down the results.

Fine-Tuning Your Diet

After you perform the test, if your pH is too high or too low, omit the acid- or alkaline-forming foods from your diet until another pH test shows that your body's pH is within a normal range. Then you can add a few of those foods back into your diet to determine what kind of diet is healthful for you. On that subject, it's now time to discuss delicious organic foods, nature's best medicine.

Why Organic Foods Are Better for Your Hormones and Overall Health

As I mentioned earlier, conventionally grown produce is tainted with pesticides, and the soil the produce grows in is heavily sprayed with toxic herbicides. The Environmental Protection Agency (EPA) has researched pesticides used in conventional agriculture and found them to contain more than 107 active ingredients that are known or probable carcinogens. I know this is disturbing, but you can avoid exposure to these poisons by eating organically.

Furthermore, according to the latest research, about 2.2 billion pounds of pesticides are used in America every year—about 8 pounds for every man, woman, and child. Some of the most severely pesticide-tainted are foods that we eat most often, such as coffee, strawberries, peanut butter, raisins, apples, milk, and cereal.

Medical research has found a link between the increase in the use of pesticides and the rise in breast cancer among American women, most likely because pesticides exert powerful estrogenic effects that lead to cancer. As I stressed in the last chapter, one of the best ways to balance hormones naturally—and protect your health—is by eating organically.

Some organic foods are more expensive than conventionally grown produce. But the extra cost of organic food is definitely justified by the nutritional benefits and the lack of toxic pesticides. If organic is not an option for you, then it's vital that you wash away as many of the pesticides, toxins, and parasites as possible. Directions for this are in part 3, which also contains delicious recipes.

From a nutritional perspective, conventionally grown produce is lower in minerals than organic produce is. This is partly because organic soil is much richer in healthful microorganisms and minerals, since no pesticides or herbicides have depleted it. Several studies have shown that organic food contains far more minerals that are crucial for your health, such as calcium, chromium, magnesium, and selenium, than conventionally grown food contains. I have had patients with PMS, allergies, asthma, eczema, chemical sensitivities, and so on, who report great improvement—and, in some cases, complete reversal—after they were on my program, which included eating organic foods for just a few months.

To ensure that you're buying organic food, look for the words Certified Organic or USDA Organic on the package.

Genetically Engineered Foods

Yet another compelling reason to eat organically is to avoid genetically engineered foods, also known as genetically modified organisms (GMOs). Did you know that 70 percent of the food on grocery store shelves is genetically modified? According to research by the Organic Consumers Association, at least 60 percent of processed foods contain ingredients derived from genetically engineered soybeans alone!

Other popular GMO foods are even sold in some health food stores. I call GMO products Frankenstein Foods and here is why.

GMOs are living organisms that have had their DNA or genetic structure reconfigured by the insertion of an alien gene, to give them traits that make them more economically viable from a seed manufacturer's or an industrial farmer's standpoint. These traits include cold tolerance, herbicide resistance, or the ability to destroy insects that eat it. Genetic engineering is presently performed on plants, vegetables, fruits, seeds, and animals. (I hope this is never done on human beings.) Multinational agribusiness behemoths like Monsanto and Dow Chemical are leading the GMO food industry. After manipulating and patenting the genes of a seed, these companies then sell the seeds around the world and acquire a hefty market share.

A typical example of a GMO food is the cold-resistant tomato that a seed company made by inserting a flounder gene into its genetic makeup. The main problems with eating foods grown from sci-fi seeds like these are

- Testing on how GMO foods affect humans has barely begun; therefore, it is unknown whether they are safe to eat.
- Genetic material can now be transferred between species that would never, ever breed in nature. (When was the last time you saw a tomato and a flounder mating?)
- GMO science is so experimental and imprecise that its effects on adults, children, and developing fetuses are unknown.
- The virus that is used to alter the genetic makeup of the food could possibly breed new viruses that cause diseases, including incurable ones.
- The U.S. government does not require GMO foods to be labeled, although in Japan and most nations in the European Union, GMO labeling is compulsory.

This means that we in the United States can never be sure when we're buying or eating GMO foods. Even if you buy produce and packaged goods like soy milk at a health food store, you have no guarantee that you're eating non-GMOs, unless it's specifically labeled "non-GMO" or "made with non-GMOs."

This last point brings us to one of the many potential nightmares served up by GMOs. Imagine that you're severely allergic to all fish. You unwittingly eat a bowl of tomato soup made from GMO tomatoes containing that previously mentioned flounder gene. Will you experience a mild allergy or experience a life-threatening reaction that requires emergency room care? More to the point, will this damage your health in the short term, the long term, or both?

Long-term studies on humans who eat GMOs have never been done. For this and other reasons, the British Medical Association and many leading scientists around the world have demanded a moratorium on the sale and the consumption of GMO foods until further research is completed.

GMO foods routinely turn up in my patients' cupboards and refrigerators. Space limitations prevent me from supplying a complete list of GMO foods in our midst, but here's a brief list of some common ones to raise your awareness about which foods to pitch from your pantry.

Aspartame, also called NutraSweet: Flavors diet soft drinks, candy, chewing gum, children's vitamins, and medicines. It's frequently found in low-fat cookies, low-fat jelly, jam, and diet yogurt.

Splenda: The dextrose in this popular chemical sweetener is derived from genetically engineered corn.

Canola: This plant oil is a major ingredient in salad dressings, cookies, snack foods, margarine, soy cheeses, and many frozen and fried foods.

Corn: Myriad foods in the typical American diet are filled with corn derivatives. These include high fructose corn syrup, cornstarch, corn oil, and corn flour.

Products that often contain GMOs made from corn include tortillas and tortilla chips, infant formula, baby food, cornbread mixes, fried foods, powdered sugar, enriched white flour, pasta, soda, and the list goes on. In addition to dextrose, sugars such as glucose, maltose, sucrose, and sugars used in canned fruit and soft drinks are all made with products derived from GMO corn. Common thickeners like xanthan gum, also known as E415, come from corn sugar and are used to thicken ice cream, salad dressings, candy, frostings, and more.

Now that you have a taste of the documented, as well as unknown, dangers lurking in GMO foods, I hope you'll consider the extra money spent on organic foods an investment in your health. Eating organically may very well help you save on doctor and hospital bills in the future. All of my patients, children and adults, thrive on organic foods.

Also, like Julia at the beginning of this chapter, they start to thrive after they cut out unhealthful fats and begin to eat the right kind of fats on a daily basis. Here's the lowdown on the right kind of fats.

Good Fats and Bad Fats

Since the widely popular Atkins Diet allows adherents to consume up to two-thirds of their calories from fat (more than double the usual recommendation), many people have concluded that it's healthful to eat animal fats in abundance. The truth is, there are good fats and bad fats, and you need to know which ones will help you and your hormones achieve optimum wellness.

It's also vital that you reduce your fat intake to less than 30 percent of your total daily calories. If you're adhering to a 2,000-calorie diet, that translates into a maximum of 65 grams of fat per day. In broad strokes, here's what you need to know about good and bad fats so that you can improve your hormone health, while reducing your risk for heart disease and other illnesses.

Bad Fats

Saturated Fat

To begin with, saturated fat, from animal and dairy products, should account for less than 10 percent of your daily calories. Multiple studies from around the world confirm that high intakes of saturated fat derived from animal sources are connected to high levels of blood cholesterol. Specifically, research indicates that saturated fat limits the effectiveness of LDL receptors on cells so that cholesterol piles up in the bloodstream. This is bad news for your cardiovascular system.

Saturated fat is found in all animal foods, such as meat, poultry, eggs, and dairy products. It's also present in coconuts, which are 92 percent saturated fat. The saturated fat in coconut oil is far more healthful for you, however, than the kind found in animal fats. Research has shown that natural coconut fat in the diet leads to a normalization of body lipids (or body fats), protects against alcohol damage to the liver, and improves the immune system's anti-inflammatory response.

Coconut oil is unusually rich in short- and medium-chain fatty acids. The healing potential of lauric acid, the major fatty acid from the fat of the coconut, has captivated researchers and nutritionists alike. This is due to its antibacterial, antiviral, and antiprotozoal functions.

Dried or creamed coconut is about 69 percent fat. Full coconut milk is approximately 24 percent fat. Approximately 50 percent of the fatty acids in coconut fat are lauric acid. Lauric acid is a medium-chain fatty acid, which possesses the additional beneficial power of transforming into monolaurin in the human body.

Monolaurin is an antibacterial, antiviral, and antiprotozoal substance that the body uses to destroy lipid-coated viruses such as HIV, herpes, and influenza, and various pathogenic bacteria and protozoa such as giardia lamblia, which taints many streams and rivers around the world.

The food industry has long known that the functional properties of coconut oil are far superior to those of other commercially available oils. In the United States, however, during the 1980s and 1990s, the commercial interests of the U.S. domestic fats and oils industry, with their anti–saturated fat agenda, succeeded at discouraging the consumption of coconut oil.

Eating raw young white coconut is your best way to enjoy this wonder food, and you can buy it at Asian markets and health food stores. If it's challenging for you to find coconut, using coconut oil is the next best thing. You can add this to your diet by using it exclusively when you cook or sauté. Because coconut oil is a completely saturated fat, it never forms dangerously unhealthy trans-fatty acids.

A diet high in saturated fats from animal sources negatively affects your health by damaging your arteries, brain cells, and genes, while also contributing to obesity. Saturated fats also stimulate the formation of inflammation molecules, which are known to promote various diseases. Eating a diet high in saturated fats, such as those found in red meat, is correlated with an increased risk of heart disease, cancer, and Alzheimer's, as well as diabetes.

Different types of saturated fats affect blood cholesterol in different ways. For instance, the saturated fat in dairy products raises cholesterol more than the saturated fat in meat does. You may be glad to know that the saturated fat in chocolate (called stearic acid) does not raise blood cholesterol levels.

Trans Fats

Trans-fatty acids are found in processed and fried foods. Trans fats undergo a chemical process wherein hydrogen atoms are added to liquid vegetable oils. While food manufacturers love hydrogenation because it makes vegetable oils more solid and gives their products flavor, there is a downside for you, the consumer. Hydrogenation destroys the essential fatty acids that you need to obtain from vegetable oils. Even worse, the dangerous trans fats that are created increase your bad cholesterol (LDL cholesterol) and decrease your good (HDL cholesterol) levels. A diet high in trans fats is heavily implicated in heart disease. *Warning:* Trans fats are much worse for you than saturated fats are.

As much as 40 percent of the fat in foods such as commercial snack crackers, cake frosting, margarine, cookies, fried fast foods, french fries, doughnuts, and pastries is in the form of hydrogenated oils. I have long referred to this artery-clogging gunk as "death oil," and extensive research supports the accuracy of my moniker. The authoritative Nurses' Health Study found that women who had the highest intake of trans fats had a 50 percent higher risk of heart disease than did women who ate the least. You can avoid eating trans fats altogether by reading label ingredients carefully. Key words to scan for are "partially hydrogenated vegetable oils" or "shortening." If you see these, throw the product away, or put it back on the store shelf!

Many people who choose to eat margarine made with hydrogenated oil, instead of eating butter, mistakenly believe that the

margarine is more healthful. I suggest substituting both with alternatives such as olive oil, walnut butter, hemp butter, or almond butter.
These are all delicious and flavor-packed, with the added bonus of
being great for your body. Find them at your health food store or
check out the Resource Guide of this book.

Good Fats

Polyunsaturated Fats

These include omega-3 and omega-6 polyunsaturated fats. Omega-3
polyunsaturated fats are present in fish and seafood, flaxseed, and
walnut oil. These fats are often called "the good fats." Omega-6
polyunsaturated fats are in all vegetable oils, including canola, sunflower, safflower, corn, and sesame. Bear in mind that replacing saturated fat in your diet with polyunsaturates will help to lower your
cholesterol.

Foods that are rich in healthful omega-3 fats, such as salmon, tuna,
olive oil, and flaxseed oil, inhibit inflammation. The two essential
fatty acids, alpha-linolenic acid (ALA) and linoleic acid (LA), that are
found in omega-3 type fats also protect your cell membranes by
upgrading your body's resistance to allergens and illness. ALA and
LA have been scientifically validated as helping to promote optimal
health, and they serve as a treatment for more than sixty health ailments. For instance, essential fatty acids help to balance hormones
that are responsible for fibrocystic breast disease. Studies have shown
flaxseed oil to be extremely beneficial: it helps to balance estrogen
during menopause, lowers cholesterol, soothes arthritic inflammation, and helps to treat multiple sclerosis.

Healthful omega-3 fats are also found in evening primrose and
borage oil. (Borage is an annual European herb with an extensive
medicinal history. Its leaves are eaten as salad greens or cooked
like spinach.)

As it happens, the highest quality of omega-3 fats are those found
in fish. That's because the omega-3 in fish is high in two fatty acids
that are crucial to human health, DHA and EPA. These two fatty
acids are pivotal in preventing heart disease, cancer, and many other
diseases. DHA is particularly essential for health, as it is the primary

structural fatty acid in the gray matter of your brain and the retina of your eyes. (I know it's hard to believe, but 60 percent of the brain is fat, even in supermodels!) DHA also ensures the optimal flexibility of nerve cell membranes that are essential for transmitting electrical signals from one brain cell to another, as well as to the rest of the body.

DHA helps you to feel and function at your best; an ongoing supply of it is necessary for proper brain function throughout life. While the average American diet is low in DHA, fatty fish, meats, and eggs are primary DHA sources. Vegetarians, people on low-fat diets, or individuals who take cholesterol-lowering drugs are particularly susceptible to DHA deficiency.

DHA deficiency is associated with certain conditions that are common in perimenopause. These include memory loss, changes in disposition, and other neurological conditions. Researchers have found that DHA supplementation helps to prevent depression and coronary artery disease, plus Alzheimer's disease and memory loss in the elderly. It also reduces symptoms associated with attention deficit hyperactivity disorder (ADHD).

If you're prone to moody PMS episodes or have a family history of coronary disease, you may be intrigued to know that polyunsaturated essential fatty acids also appear to play a pivotal role in positive moods and heart health. U.S. researchers reported in a 2004 issue of the *European Journal of Clinical Nutrition* that the presence of hostility in an individual predicts both the development and the manifestation of coronary disease. In one study, the consumption of either DHA or fish, which is high in omega-3 fatty acids, was associated with lower odds of a person having high hostility. Researchers now link inadequate intake of DHA and EPA in pregnant women to premature birth and low birth weight babies and to hyperactivity in children.

Both omega-3 and omega-6 are essential for human health. The typical American, however, consumes far too many omega-6 fats, while consuming very low levels of omega-3. The ideal ratio of omega-6 to omega-3 fats is 1:1. Over millions of years, our ancestors evolved on this ratio. Today, though, our ratio of omega-6 to omega-3 averages from 20:1 to 50:1! That spells danger. Avoid or limit corn, canola, safflower, and sunflower oils.

Friendly Fat Facts

As a certified clinical nutritionist, I've helped thousands of people achieve radiant health through proper nutrition. I can assure you that following a diet that's high in essential fatty acids and low in animal fats is the most healthful way to maintain proper hormone balance and the overall health of organs and body systems. Eliminate red meat and supplement your daily diet with one to two tablespoons of oils that are rich in essential fatty acids, such as organic flaxseed or borage oil. Borage oil is a superb source of gammalinolenic acid (GLA) and is a delicious option in salad dressings, sauces, stir fries, and so on.

Each individual needs a different amount of fats, so it's impossible to provide a blanket recommendation for daily fat intake. Generally speaking, humans benefit from eating 20 to 30 percent of their daily calories as fats from vegetable sources, because a lack of essential fatty acids appears to promote degenerative diseases. Symptoms of essential fatty acid deficiency include PMS, migraines, high cholesterol or triglycerides, hypertension, eczema and other skin disorders, immune disorders, arthritis, and inflammatory disease.

Surveys indicate that at least 80 percent of people in the United States are deficient in the essential fatty acids, which may help to explain why so many Americans suffer from the previously listed conditions. Mass commercial refinement of fats and oils (and of processed foods that contain them) has effectively eliminated the essential fatty acids from our diet, which contributes to this deficiency. Therefore, we need to eat organic, unrefined oils.

Omega-3 fats are typically found in flaxseed oil, walnut oil, and fish oil. The goal is to increase your intake of the omega-3 fats found in fish oil and reduce your intake of omega-6 fats. Sadly, though, eating fresh fish, whether from the ocean, lakes, streams, or fish farms, puts your health at risk. Mercury and PCB levels in all fish have now hit dangerously high concentrations around the world, and the health risks of mercury and PCBs far outweigh the omega-3 benefits of eating fish. While mercury can kill brain cells and other types of neurons, PCBs also exert various toxic effects.

There are 209 types of PCBs, which are chemicals used in various industries such as electrical products. Some PCBs act like hormones, while others act like nerve poisons; still others alter major systems in the body, such as the immune, nervous, and enzyme systems. In 2004, the U.S. Food and Drug Administration (FDA) advised that pregnant women, women of childbearing age, nursing mothers, and young children avoid eating certain kinds of fish that may contain high levels of methyl mercury, such as shark, swordfish, king mackerel, and tile fish.

Routine consumption of fish oil, however, is highly encouraged as a key ingredient in improving your health. Fish oil contains the highest levels of the best omega-3 fats—those with EPA and DHA fatty acids—and, because it's in a pure form, does not pose the mercury risk of eating fresh fish.

Monounsaturated Fats

Monounsaturated fats found in olive oil, canola oil, and peanut oil have scant effect on cholesterol levels. But when you eat these instead of saturated fat, you lower your levels of blood cholesterol. The next time you crave some fat, satisfy yourself by eating a salad dressed with organic olive oil and vinegar, instead of cheese and crackers.

The Most Healthful Oils

Organic flaxseed oil tops the list of nourishing oils. Many people consider flaxseed oil the answer to the essential fatty acids dilemma. Oil extracted from flaxseeds is a health wonder because it contains both essential fatty acids: alpha-linolenic, an omega-3 fatty acid, and linoleic acid, an omega-6 fatty acid, in significant amounts. Flaxseed oil is the world's richest source of omega-3 fatty acids, at a fabulous 57 percent (more than two times the amount of omega-3 fatty acids in fish oils).

Omega-3 fatty acids have been extensively studied for their beneficial effects on the following conditions: arthritis, cancer, high cholesterol levels, heart pain (angina), high blood pressure, multiple sclerosis, psoriasis, eczema, stroke, and heart attack. The high content of omega-3 fatty acids in flaxseed oil is just one of its positive attributes.

The essential fatty acids that are combined in flaxseed oil have been proven to help regulate the body's fatty acid metabolism. Fat metabolism is as important, if not more important, than our body's metabolism of proteins and carbohydrates, as indicated by today's epidemic of fat-related degenerative diseases, such as vascular disease and strokes.

Essential fatty acids in flaxseed oil are converted to hormonelike substances known as prostaglandins and are key players in managing numerous key bodily functions. These include steroid production and hormone synthesis; inflammation, pain, and swelling; pressure in the eye, the joints, or the blood vessels; gastrointestinal, arterial, ear, and heart functions; water retention; blood-clotting ability; allergic response; and rheumatoid arthritis. Without the essential fatty acids, the building blocks of prostaglandins, the body is destined to have fat-metabolism malfunctions and problems in regulating the bodily functions, as cited earlier.

Organic Olive Oil

The greatest example of monounsaturated fat is olive oil, which is a natural juice that preserves the taste, the aroma, the vitamins, and the properties of the olive fruit. Olive oil is the only vegetable oil that can be consumed freshly pressed from the fruit. Olive oil is a prime component of the Mediterranean diet.

About 30 percent of the calories of the Mediterranean diet come from fat, and the majority of fat calories come from olive oil. The cancer rate among Italian women is 30 percent lower than among American women; their risk of heart disease is markedly lower, as well. Olive oil's beneficial health effects are due to its high content of monounsaturated fatty acids and antioxidative substances.

Studies have shown that olive oil offers protection against heart disease by controlling LDL ("bad") cholesterol levels, while raising HDL (the "good" cholesterol) levels. No other naturally produced oil has such a large amount of monounsaturated fat as olive oil does.

Olive oil is very easily digested and helps stomach conditions such as ulcers and gastritis. Studies have found that olive oil stimulates the secretion of bile and pancreatic hormones much more effectively than prescription drugs do. Eating olive oil on a daily basis appears to help lower the risk of developing gallstones.

Please disregard any hype you have heard about the supposed superiority of canola (rapeseed) oil over olive oil, due to its concentration of monounsaturated fatty acids. Olive oil, especially extra virgin olive oil, is chemically and nutritionally superior.

Olive Oil and Your Health

Studies have shown that people who consumed 25 milliliters (mL), or about 2 tablespoons, of virgin olive oil daily for one week showed less oxidation of LDL cholesterol and higher levels of antioxidant compounds, particularly phenols, in the blood. All types of olive oil are sources of monounsaturated fat, but extra virgin olive oil, from the first pressing of the olives, contains the highest levels of antioxidants—namely, vitamin E and phenols—because it is less refined. For optimum health and cardiac protection, I recommend that you buy extra virgin oil.

Some research suggests that including olive oil in your diet may also help to prevent colon cancer. In a Spanish study, results showed that rats fed supplemental olive oil had a lower risk of colon cancer than did those fed safflower oil–supplemented diets. In fact, the rats that ate olive oil had colon cancer rates almost as low as those fed fish oil, which several studies have previously connected to reduced colon cancer risk.

Now that we've covered the ups and downs of fats, which comprise a hefty 33 percent of the American diet, let's turn to carbohydrates.

Good Carbs, Bad Carbs

Carbohydrates are a controversial diet topic, mainly because we eat so much of them—and because excess carbs turn to sugar in the body and then are stored as fat. If you're wondering what exactly is a carbohydrate, let me explain. A carbohydrate is the sugar, the starch, or the fiber in a food. Starch is merely the storage form of sugar. Generally speaking, carbohydrates are found in every fruit, vegetable, or grain.

Although you benefit from eating carbs in the form of vegetables or fruits because they contain micronutrients such as vitamins and minerals, the same cannot be said for other carb-rich foods. Many unrefined foods and processed foods consist mainly of carbs: sugar, flour, and cereal grains such as rice, corn, oats, and wheat. Also carb-heavy are all the foods made from these things, such as breads, cereals, cakes, chips, pasta, rice cakes, and so forth. Except for their starch or sugar content, these foods are nutritionally weak, unless they're vitamin-fortified.

Unfortunately, research shows that women are eating far more carbs than they did thirty years ago. According to a 2004 U.S. Centers for Disease Control and Prevention (CDC) study, a woman's average caloric intake topped out at 1,542 calories in 1971. By 2000, the average woman ate 355 more calories daily than in 1971.

According to the CDC epidemiologist and study author Jacqueline Wright, most of the calorie increase comes from a hike in carbohydrates. Rather than coming from fruits and vegetables, which are high in amino acids, the building blocks of protein, minerals, and health-enhancing micronutrients, the bad carbs that women are eating today lurk inside nutritionally deficient filler foods, such as cookies, bagels, chips, pasta, and sodas.

The main problem with eating bad carbs from refined grains such as white flour or white rice is that they are quickly digested and rapidly turn to sugar in your body, hence into fat. Refined grains are also less nutritionally dense than whole grains are. On the other hand, the complex carbohydrates in organic whole grains, such as brown rice, quinoa, spelt, millet, or buckwheat, are nutritionally richer and are digested far more slowly than the carbs in refined grains are. Complex carbohydrates are essential for energy; if you're exercising a lot, incorporate organic whole grains into your diet.

Now we need to take a look at sugars, which on average make up 25 percent of what we eat.

Good Sugars, Bad Sugars, and Synthetic Sugar Substitutes

Most of us eat sugar in the form of white sugar. This heavily refined product undergoes thirty-two different processes, including bleaching. I refer to this sweet stuff as "little white death crystals." You may recall that eating too much of any form of sugar can lead to adrenal exhaustion and hormone imbalances, not to mention that it can raise your risk of developing diabetes. These in turn can aggravate PMS and perimenopausal symptoms, while leading to mood disorders and a host of other problematic conditions that sap your energy and make life more challenging than it needs to be.

I'm not opposed to eating sweetened foods, but for health reasons, I recommend using only organic agave syrup or stevia. Why? Both of these unrefined substances provide wonderful sweetness without the empty calories, weight gain, and adrenal strain associated with other forms of sugar.

Take agave syrup, for example. It's produced by steeping milled brown rice in a special plant-derived enzyme preparation. This process transforms the steamed grain into a smooth-flavored, deliciously sweet syrup. Agave syrup is hypoallergenic, is gluten free, and is made without the use of any cane or beet sugars, corn syrups, or other refined sweeteners of any kind. You can use agave syrup just as you would white sugar, only you'll need less. Two tablespoons add up to a modest 120 calories, and you can find it in health food stores.

As for stevia, this contains zero calories, is safe for diabetics, and has been used for centuries in South American cultures. It is derived from a perennial shrub of the aster family. Although it is 300 times sweeter than sugar, the herb can be used safely by diabetics. Stevia contains niacin, magnesium, potassium, and vitamin C. Research indicates that it may reduce cavities by slowing the growth of dental plaque, in marked contrast to tooth-decaying white sugar. You can find stevia in health food stores, specialty markets, and many gourmet shops.

I give rave reviews to both agave syrup and stevia. Although many sweeteners are sold at markets and health food stores, I never recommend using any of the following because they will affect blood sugar: barley malt, brown rice syrup, date sugar, fruit juice concentrate, fructose, honey, maple sugar, maple syrup, molasses, sucanat (made from organic blackstrap molasses and evaporated cane juice), or turbinado sugar.

Lest you think that sugar substitutes are a healthful alternative, check out the following case history of one of my patients who was hooked on them.

Kathy's hormone saliva tests indicated that she was in adrenal exhaustion. I questioned her about her diet. She swore that she was on the endocrine-rebuilding diet that I had given her and that she was eating lots of healthful organic food. She said that she consumed neither caffeine nor sugar but drank lots of Diet Coke because she didn't like water. What's more, she used Splenda for a sweetener. Kathy had been on my diet for three weeks and still didn't feel better.

I explained to Kathy that the five sodas she drank each day contained sugar substitutes, as well as other chemicals that age the body and make the adrenal glands, the pancreas, the kidneys, and the liver work especially hard. After I mentioned reports on Splenda-induced allergic reactions, Kathy finally understood that Splenda is a chemical and that switching to agave syrup and stevia could give her a chance to lighten up.

One week later, Kathy enthused about how much better she felt—more energetic than she had in many months. Her menopause symptoms were gone, and she plans to use natural sweeteners forever.

Let me dish out some facts on synthetic sweeteners, beginning with Splenda. This is sucralose, or chlorinated sugar. It is not a friendly substance to the body. Sucralose can account for health problems such as atrophy of the thymus gland, the kidneys, and the liver; miscarriage; low fetal weight; and increased glycosylated hemoglobin. There are also reports of Splenda causing severe allergic reactions, including breathing problems, large welts, and rashes.

As for aspartame, also known as NutraSweet, this contains the amino acid phenylalanine, which can clamp up blood vessels, causing headaches. You need to eliminate this from your diet as well, because aspartame has been proven to block the formation of serotonin, the feel-good neurotransmitter that you need in order to maintain a positive mood. If you think that consuming NutraSweet may be contributing to your PMS or mood problems, this is another compelling reason to give it up immediately.

Salt, Minerals, and Trace Elements

Did you know that studies indicate that most Americans overdose on salt every day? Some research indicates that we eat two teaspoons of salt (4,600 mg sodium) each day, almost ten times more than we need! While it's true that we need salt to live, we don't need that much. I recommend that you ditch table salt altogether in favor of Celtic sea salt, organic tamari sauce, or organic ponzu sauce.

Copious research indicates that most people in the United States have at least one hidden deficiency of a major mineral, such as calcium or magnesium. Even if you have a "balanced" or healthful diet and take supplements, your body could still lack vital minerals and trace elements. It's impossible to thoroughly cover all of the minerals and trace minerals here; however, locating this information is quite easy, as many books have been written on the subject. Now, we'll discuss a few essential vital minerals that critically affect hormone and bone health.

Magnesium

I find that many people are magnesium deficient, mostly because of their diet, as well as their alcohol, drug, and caffeine intake, all of which cause mineral loss. Magnesium plays an important role in regulating the neuromuscular activity of the heart. It also maintains normal heart rhythm and is necessary for proper calcium and vitamin C metabolism. Finally, it converts blood sugar into energy.

Silica

Silica (which is a silicon compound) is the most abundant element in the earth's strata. The human body, if it weighs in at around 150 pounds, would contain approximately one and one quarter ounces of silica, a quantity that far exceeds the amounts of other important minerals such as iron. Both iron and silica are essential in facilitating the ongoing metabolic processes that are vital to life. In 1939, the Nobel Prize winner for chemistry, Professor Adolf Butenant, proved that life as we know it cannot exist without silica.

According to research conducted at Columbia University in 1972, silica is an essential nutrient and must be continuously supplied from food sources. Hormonal disturbances in the human organism are often due to a calcium-magnesium imbalance. Several studies have shown that silica can restore this delicate balance. Silica also aids in the assimilation of phosphorus and is considered a catalyst in the body's utilization of other natural elements.

Silica is found throughout the body. It reinforces the body's membranes, the tissues, the arterial walls, the throat walls, the uterine lining, the walls of the digestive tract, the tendons, the spinal and cerebral dura mater, the nails, and the skin.

Silica is necessary for the formation of collagen in bones and connective tissue. It helps to prevent osteoporosis and is vital in the early stages of bone formation because it aids in calcium absorption. The men in our lives can also benefit from taking silica, especially men who suffer from lack of tone in the testicles. Moreover, a silica-rich diet is effective against impotence. In addition, women who have cysts in the vagina and health concerns regarding the mammary glands, such as hardened glands or pus generation, can be helped by taking silica.

The tissues in the body are made alkaline by silica, which can contribute to your developing a quick, agile, lean, and flexible body. Silica unites with sulfur to create healthy hair and nails. People who suffer from ovarian or menstrual complications, mental and emotional imbalances, and nervous system disorders will also benefit from silica.

People over age fifty have reported good results from the use of silica: joint elasticity and eyesight are enhanced, the complexion is improved, and varicose veins are reduced. Studies reveal that nations with the lowest cancer rates are known for having diets high in silica.

Silica is an essential partner in creating strong, healthy bones and aids in the absorption of all minerals, including calcium and magnesium. You can purchase homeopathic silica, as well as a silica supplement that may contain the herb horsetail. (The chief medicinal property of horsetail is its high silica content.)

The best dietary source of silica is whole grains, because much of the silica in our diets is lost in the refining process. Silica is necessary for maintaining flexible arteries and plays a major role in the preventing of cardiovascular disease. Furthermore, silica is used widely to counteract the effects of aluminum on the body, thus making it important in the prevention of Alzheimer's disease.

Unfortunately, silica levels in our bodies decrease as we age, so we need to consume more silica-rich foods. Maintaining a youthful, sexy body requires silica, because it stimulates the immune system and inhibits the aging process. Boron, calcium, magnesium, manganese, and potassium help to promote the efficient utilization of silica.

Beneficial Boron

Over the last decade, we have acquired a much greater understanding of cellular communication and the balance of nutrients in our bodies. We have embraced the discoveries of nutrients such as coenzyme Q10, acetyl L-carnitine, alpha-lipoic acid, lycopene, selenium, and gamma tocopherol—just a few examples of new players in the symphony of good health. We can now add boron, a trace element nutrient, to the orchestra.

A large number of experiments conducted on people show that boron is vitally involved in bone metabolism. It's well accepted that calcium and magnesium are important constituents or building blocks of healthy bone. In situations where the body receives an adequate supply of calcium but has deficient magnesium resources, boron seems to actively substitute for magnesium during the process of bone formation. Under such conditions, the concentration of boron within bone tissue increases.

Boron has the ability to reduce the urinary excretion of calcium and magnesium. It preserves calcium in the body, while decreasing urinary losses of calcium, through its actions on the kidneys. The calcium-preserving effect of boron becomes pronounced when dietary magnesium is low. Think of boron as your personal bodyguard, which preserves calcium and magnesium when your body is nutritionally stressed. Some research reveals that boron also alleviates joint discomfort and preserves cognitive function.

A boron deficiency seems to influence calcium and magnesium metabolism and affects the composition, the structure, and the strength of bone, leading to changes similar to those seen in osteoporosis. This is likely due to decreased absorption and the increased excretion of calcium and magnesium. A boron deficiency, combined with a magnesium deficiency, appears especially damaging in cases of osteoporosis. Due to its effects on calcium and magnesium metabolism, a boron deficiency may also contribute to the formation of kidney stones. A boron deficiency seems to decrease mental alertness as well.

Sources of boron include noncitrus fruits like dried prunes, plums, grapes, and raisins; nuts such as almonds and peanuts; red wine; and coffee. Boron supplements are available in health food stores.

The Good News on Calcium

Because calcium is such a controversial mineral and is so critical to bone health and the prevention of osteoporosis, a few words about this mineral are in order. One of the most important minerals in the body, calcium is also the most abundant mineral found in the human body, constituting about 1.5 to 2 percent of our body weight. Our bones contain most of this calcium (98 percent), and the rest is split between our teeth (1 percent) and other tissues and the circulatory system.

Scientific research in Germany and elsewhere indicates that the form of calcium known as calcium orotate is far superior to any other form of calcium in promoting bone growth, bone hardening, and bone density. This is because calcium orotate, unlike other forms of calcium, can penetrate complex cell membranes and is metabolized in cartilage.

You can find calcium orotate, minerals, and trace minerals in health food stores and on the Internet. I'd also like to add that research indicates that prevention of bone loss can be achieved through regular exercise, combined with eating dark-green leafy vegetables such as swiss chard, spinach, and beet and dandelion greens.

I suggest a daily dose of calcium orotate, depending on your body's individual needs. Research and my own experience indicate that women seem more willing to change their diets than to exercise. For that reason, you must make a conscious, regular effort and apply some discipline if you want to increase your bone density and reverse or prevent mineral loss. If you follow the detoxification plan in chapter 3 and drink a daily glass of the revitalizing vegetable juice from that chapter, your mineral needs will be well met.

The following Mineral Self-Assessment Test will give you more insight into what your symptoms are telling you about your body's mineral balance.

Mineral Self-Assessment Test

Check all that apply to you now or recently.

Group A

- ☐ achy joint(s)
- ☐ a tendency to get kidney stones
- ☐ heel spurs or other bone spurs
- ☐ twitches or facial tics
- ☐ receding gums
- ☐ gingivitis or pyorrhea
- ☐ insomnia
- ☐ spinal curvature
- ☐ premenstrual distress
- ☐ osteoporosis or Paget's disease
- ☐ bursitis or painful tendons
- ☐ cramps—in legs at night, during menstruation, and so on
- ☐ dental caries (cavities)
- ☐ hypertension/irritability
- ☐ arthritic conditions (gnarled knuckles, etc.)

Group B

- ☐ irregular heartbeats
- ☐ constipation
- ☐ hyperactivity
- ☐ cold extremities or simply just feeling cold a lot
- ☐ heart disease

Group C

- ☐ pale and anemic-looking
- ☐ recurrent yeast infections/candida
- ☐ parents or grandparents who had cancer
- ☐ liver problems, particularly cirrhosis
- ☐ muscular weakness and imbalance
- ☐ a smoking habit
- ☐ residence in a humid, high-rainfall climate
- ☐ chronic tiredness
- ☐ anyone in your birth family with cystic fibrosis
- ☐ heart disease or family history of heart problems
- ☐ a strict vegetarian diet (no meat, eggs, milk)
- ☐ low resistance to infection
- ☐ family history of cataracts

Group D

- ☐ chronic tiredness
- ☐ frequent urination
- ☐ impotence
- ☐ menstrual distress
- ☐ alcoholism (Are you in recovery?)
- ☐ dizziness upon standing or getting up
- ☐ always thirsty, or never thirsty
- ☐ infertility
- ☐ liver problems (difficulty with digestion)
- ☐ a parent or a grandparent who's had Alzheimer's
- ☐ a family problem with hypoglycemia or diabetes

Group E

- ☐ premature graying of the hair
- ☐ wrinkles
- ☐ thin skin
- ☐ liver cirrhosis
- ☐ anemia
- ☐ sagging skin
- ☐ any family member who's had an aneurysm
- ☐ arthritic conditions

Group F

- [ ] a tendency to get infections
- [ ] residence in a polluted urban area
- [ ] a tendency to be anxious or nervous
- [ ] poor short-term memory
- [ ] a smoking habit, small or large

- [ ] a cold or a flu every year
- [ ] shallow breathing
- [ ] muscles that ache a long time after working out
- [ ] bruises that take a long time to heal
- [ ] sealed house or office with AC/heat year-round

Group G

- [ ] dry, brittle hair
- [ ] dry, brittle finger- and toe-nails
- [ ] poor skin quality
- [ ] poor calcium utilization
- [ ] arterial disease

- [ ] voracious appetite
- [ ] liver abscess
- [ ] urinary problems
- [ ] pyloritis
- [ ] nervous prostration due to excessive work or passion

Count up your checkmarks. If you checked 2 or more in a group, check off its corresponding group below: you may have a deficiency in that mineral.

- [ ] Group A: Calcium
- [ ] Group B: Magnesium
- [ ] Group C: Selenium
- [ ] Group D: Chromium/Vanadium

- [ ] Group E: Copper
- [ ] Group F: Oxygen
- [ ] Group G: Silica

Enzymes: Powerful Keys to Healthful Nutrition

Enzymes are as essential to your diet as amino acids, good fats, plant nutrients, protein, carbohydrates, and vitamins are. Enzymes are molecular machines that are found in nature; they're made of protein and can catalyze (speed up) chemical reactions, creating new molecules. When enzymes in organisms fall below a certain level, life ceases. Most metabolic enzymes in organisms, including plants, are killed at temperatures that exceed 118 degrees Fahrenheit. This is why I recommend eating lots of raw vegetables, because their healthful enzymes are intact, which is essential for maintaining a healthy body.

Enzymes speed and regulate all chemical reactions in the body; without them, life couldn't exist. They're made in the body from proteins and are provided when we eat enzyme-rich foods. They work by changing vitamins and minerals into forms that are usable by the body. They assist in freeing nutrients from food and help to manage chemical processes, such as detoxification. Enzymes also activate various enzymes and, guess what? They activate hormones, too.

There are three major groups of biological enzymes: food enzymes, digestive enzymes, and metabolic enzymes. As much as 40 percent of the proteins made on a daily basis in the body are used to produce more than 3,000 of our enzymes. During sickness, stressful times, or dieting, the body's enzyme production can drop to low levels.

It's been confirmed that the enzyme content of foods has significantly decreased over the years as a result of processing, refining, and preservation techniques and chemicals used in the production of mass market food items. A decreased consumption of fermented and fresh foods has also lowered the average American's enzyme intake. Deficiency can result in chronic disease, accelerated aging, and premature death.

Recently, a powerful new enzyme that supports activation of many of the body's 3,000 internal enzymes was discovered. It is called nattokinase and is derived from fermented soy and the bacteria *Bacillus natto*. You can get it at health food stores. This oddly named enzyme appears to be an effective support in a wide array of health conditions. These include endometriosis, uterine fibroids, infertility, and other gynecological conditions. What's more, nattokinase also shows promise in helping hypertension, cardiovascular conditions, stroke, angina, fibromyalgia/chronic fatigue, poor healing, varicose veins, muscle spasms, and more.

Amino Acids: How They Feed Your Body and Your Hormones

Water comprises about 60 to 70 percent of our body weight, followed by amino acids, which make up 20 percent of our weight. Amino acids are the invaluable raw materials that the body uses to make muscles, hormones, enzymes, and the vital brain chemicals called neurotransmitters. Therefore, amino acids strongly influence our physical, as well as our emotional and mental, health. About five hundred kinds of amino acids have been discovered, yet only twenty kinds of these constitute our body proteins. When you eat foods such as meat, fish, or cereals, the proteins in it are first transformed into twenty kinds of amino acids and then are reassembled as proteins in the body. Of the twenty kinds of amino acids that serve as building blocks, eleven kinds can be synthesized in the human body when needed, whereas the remaining nine kinds cannot be synthesized in the body. These are called essential amino acids. "Essential" means that we must necessarily take them from our food. Although the other amino acids are called nonessential amino acids, they are also vital in making up the body. When you eat vegetables, their amino acids are absorbed by the body.

Here's a rundown of the essential amino acids that are most important to your health.

Histidine: Found abundantly in hemoglobin; used in the treatment of rheumatoid arthritis, allergic conditions, ulcers, and anemia. A deficiency can cause poor hearing.

Phenylalanine: Used by the brain to produce norepinephrine, a chemical that transmits signals between nerve cells and the brain; keeps you awake and alert; reduces hunger pangs; functions as an antidepressant; and helps to improve memory.

Lysine: Valuable for building proteins; this tends to be deficient in white flour and white rice. Lysine deficiency can lead to growth failure.

Tryptophan: Manufactures many useful components of proteins and has a calming effect on mood.

Methionine: A principal source of sulfur, which prevents disorders of the hair, the skin, and the nails. It helps to lower cholesterol levels by increasing the liver's production of lecithin; reduces liver fat and protects the kidneys; is a natural chelating agent for heavy metals; regulates the formation of ammonia and creates ammonia-free urine, which reduces bladder irritation; and influences hair follicles and promotes hair growth.

Threonine: An important constituent of collagen, elastin, and enamel protein; helps to prevent fat buildup in the liver; helps the digestive and intestinal tracts function more smoothly; and assists in metabolism and assimilation.

Valine: Promotes mental vigor, muscle coordination, and calm emotions.

Leucine and isoleucine: Provide ingredients for the manufacture of other essential biocomponents in the body, some of which are utilized to produce energy, stimulate the upper brain, and promote alertness.

To ensure that you obtain the amino acids your body needs for optimum health and hormone balance, follow the detoxification diet in the previous chapter, drink the revitalization juice, and follow the dietary and nutritional recommendations in this chapter.

Aging and Free Radicals

Free radicals are the culprits in cases of advanced aging. They are known to target the mitochondria, the power plants of our cells. Studies have shown that on a calorie-restricted diet, the accumulation of free radicals in the body is delayed and the rate of human metabolism is decreased. This potentially means that the human lifespan can be significantly extended.

While diet is certainly crucial, many herbs and nutrients can be introduced into the body to help slow down the aging process. If we are to live long enough to take advantage of new discoveries such as stem cells, which we may be able to transform into specialized cells and tissues to treat diseases and slow aging, it's critical that we protect ourselves against the risks of dying from age-related diseases today.

So what can we do about free radicals? Left unchecked, free radicals can cause extensive cell damage and contribute to a whole list of chronic diseases. Luckily, the body does have a defense system against these rogue oxidant compounds: antioxidants. Antioxidants literally mop up free radicals. We can add to the team of antioxidants our bodies produce naturally by eating fruits and vegetables.

Familiar antioxidants include vitamins E and C, the carotenoids (such as beta-carotene), selenium, and flavonoids (such as anthocyanidins, polyphenols, quercetin). All of these are readily supplied by a varied and well-balanced diet. Probably lesser known are the so-called factory-installed antioxidants produced by the body itself, including glutathione, alpha-lipoic acid, and coenzyme Q10. Following is more information about specific antioxidants:

Lipoic acid: Considered by many researchers to be the most versatile and powerful antioxidant of all. Research indicates that it confers protection against stroke and heart disease. Lipoic acid is the only antioxidant that can significantly raise levels of glutathione, another powerful antioxidant that helps to eliminate toxins from the body. Lipoic acid can recycle glutathione, which is great news for your body, because, when taken orally, glutathione is not well absorbed by the body and is therefore rendered useless. When you supplement with lipoic acid, you're also getting a good amount of glutathione in your body.

Vitamin E: Studies prove that taking this antioxidant in a mixed tocopherol form can help prevent heart disease, reduce the risk of prostate cancer, and slow the onset of Alzheimer's disease.

Vitamin C: Must be obtained through food or supplements. It has been documented as killing free radicals with great effectiveness, and it helps to maintain a strong immune system.

Coenzyme Q-10: A fat-soluble molecule that works with vitamin E to protect the fatty part of the cell from destruction by free radicals. Several studies show that Co-Q10 is a valuable supplement for people recovering from heart failure or those living with angina or high blood pressure.

Glutathione: Produced by the body from amino acids (glutamic acid, cysteine, and glycine) in your food. Glutathione is found in almost every cell in your body; it's highly effective against free radicals. At any age, low levels of this substance are correlated with premature death and disease. After age forty, our glutathione production slows down. It declines almost 20 percent by the time we are sixty. For maximum health and positive aging, you must keep high glutathione levels in your body.

Space limitations prevent me from covering all the other antioxidants that help protect your cells from free radical invasion. If you want to find out more about this topic, I suggest that you buy some books by the nutritional supplement researcher and health author Earl Mindell, Ph.D. (See the Resource Guide.)

Cutting-Edge Nutraceutical News

Imagine a compound that can tell the difference between healthy human tissue and cancer and knows how to destroy the cancer without harming the healthy cells. Artemisinin can perform this astonishing feat. It is the jewel in the crown of antioxidants. Extracted from dry leaves of the sweet wormwood plant, artemisinin is of special interest to doctors treating PMS, cramping, excessive bleeding, and other gynecological conditions.

Artemisinin is also an antimalarial agent extracted from the dry leaves of the Chinese herb *Artemisia annua* (qinghaosu or sweet wormwood). Wormwood is cultivated only in China and Vietnam and in pilot projects in Tanzania and India. It takes eight months to mature.

Artemisinin acts rapidly and potently against the malarial parasite, including some drug-resistant strains. Without significant side effects, it quickly reduces fever and lowers the blood levels of the parasite. In a malaria epidemic in the early 1990s in Vietnam, artemisinin reduced the death rate by 97 percent.

The medical literature abounds with case histories of artemisinin helping to remedy severe life-threatening conditions such as stage-4 breast cancer, skin cancer, and lung cancer. In human beings, there are very few reports of adverse effects (see the Resource Guide for articles from the Internet on artemisinin's use for cancer and information on its side effects).

Toxic side effects of wormwood can be much more severe than artemisinin; therefore, I do not recommend usage without your consulting your health-care provider. Human use of artemisinin should be considered experimental and taking artemisinin or any other drug should be approached with extreme caution and responsibility. Check with your health-care provider before using artemisinin or wormwood.

Custom Nutritional Recommendations

The following recommendations are for conditions that are common to women and are touched on throughout this book. To educate yourself further about nutritional supplements, I recommend Dr. Earl Mindell's books. (See the Resource Guide.)

Every month, I receive dozens of e-mails from women who experience heavy menstrual bleeding (menorrhagia). Although homeopathic remedies are listed in chapter 7 to control and balance this condition, I'd also like to give you a nutritional formula to try.

Nutritional Formula for Menorrhagia (Heavy Bleeding)

Vitamin C and bioflavonoids can be very effective in ameliorating this common condition. They are not easily obtained from food alone, and they work better when taken together. A daily multinutrient vitamin formula made from whole organic food is necessary, along with the following supplements.

Powdered, mineral-buffered vitamin C: 1,000–4,000 mg per day. (This form is preferable, as some people have difficulty digesting large vitamin C pills.) Divide into two or more doses to ensure constant optimal levels, as vitamin C quickly leaves the body.

Bioflavonoids: 1,500–3,500 mg per day. Take this in two or three doses. Most bioflavonoid supplements are derived from citrus fruits and are extremely safe. However, naringin, a grapefruit-derived bioflavonoid, can interact badly with several prescription medications. If you're concerned, speak with your pharmacist or ask your health food store to order a supplement that's free of grapefruit-derived bioflavonoids.

Rutin: 1,000 mg per day, is a particularly potent bioflavonoid that's derived from buckwheat. Take 500 mg twice daily.

Hormone-Balancing Nutritional Tea

Also for heavy bleeding, this delicious tea blend is loaded with vitamin C and bioflavonoids, which help to regulate menstrual flow and promote menstrual regularity. It's caffeine-free and easy to make, and you can buy ingredients in bulk at health food stores.

INGREDIENTS FOR HORMONE-BALANCING NUTRITIONAL TEA

4 cups water
2 teaspoons rose hips herb
1 teaspoon raspberry leaf
2 teaspoons blackberry leaf
¼ teaspoon orange peel
¼ teaspoon lemon peel
stevia or agave syrup (optional)

Bring the water to a boil. Add the herbs to the water and stir. Turn the heat to low and simmer for 15 minutes. Add stevia or agave syrup to sweeten if desired.

More on Hormone-Balancing Nourishment

By now, you realize what a key role nutrition plays in promoting hormonal balance. As you learned in the previous chapter, a critical step in achieving hormone health involves internal cleansing. Liver congestion can cause hormonal imbalances. If the liver is congested, it cannot fully conjugate hormones so that the body can utilize them.

Because it's important to detoxify the gallbladder, the kidneys, the blood, and the colon while you support the immune system, I recommend daily skin brushing and dry saunas two to three times weekly to help promote detoxification. When you're taking saunas, you need more essential fatty acids, so you should consume more organic ground flaxseeds, vitamin E, and B vitamins.

Nutrients for Hormonal Balance

Hormonal imbalances are often connected to various symptoms that can be treated naturally with homeopathy and good nutrition. I've prepared a list of symptoms that often accompany hormonal complaints and nutrients that can remedy these symptoms by helping to rebuild the endocrine system. These nutritional supplements can be purchased in the health food store.

Nutrients for Hormonal Balance

The following nutrients are helpful in rebuilding the endocrine system and can be purchased at any health food store.

Blood Sugar Wellness (sugar cravings)
- [ ] Alpha-lipoic acid
- [ ] Chromium picolinate
- [ ] Homeopathic Meridian Remedy for Pancreas/Spleen (low self-esteem and rejection)

Digestive Wellness
- [ ] Digestive enzyme: to digest carbohydrates, protein, and fats

Dysbiosis; Candida; Parasites
- [ ] Probiotic (good bacteria for intestines)
- [ ] Artemesia Forte (parasites)
- [ ] Caprylate complex (candida)

Vitamin and Mineral Formulas
- [ ] Women's multi made from whole food
- [ ] Vitamin C ascorbates with bioflavonoids (Since we don't manufacture vitamin C in our bodies, everyone needs to take C or eat an abundance of fruits.)
- [ ] Calcium/magnesium: orotate and citrate form, with boron
- [ ] Trace mineral complex

Immune Function: Edema, Inflammation, and Infections
- [ ] Herbal diuretic (edema)
- [ ] Wobenzym N (proteolytic enzyme)
- [ ] Glucosamine/MSM (joint/ tissue pain)
- [ ] D-mannose powder for urinary tract
- [ ] Organic olive leaf (infections)
- [ ] Organic oregano oil (infections)
- [ ] Garlic liquid or capsules (infections)
- [ ] Vitamin C combined with bioflavonoids and rutin (infections, joint/tissue repair)
- [ ] Mushroom combination: reishi, maitake, and so on
- [ ] Gallbladder/Liver /Kidney Flush Kit

Meridian/Emotional Balance and Healing
- [ ] MetaWellness Home Study Course (see Resource Guide)
- [ ] Homeopathic meridian remedies (see Resource Guide)

Heart Wellness
- [ ] Co-Q10
- [ ] Homeopathic remedies

Hormone and Cortisol Balance

☐ Phosphatidyl choline (use for low adrenal cortisol levels)

☐ Phosphatidyl serine (revitalizes nerve cells; use for high adrenal cortisol levels and for mental clarity)

☐ Natural mixed vitamin E, 800 mg or more

☐ Sho Wu Pill (adrenal stress and hair loss)

☐ Thyroid: kelp, amino acid (L-tyrosine), homeopathic remedies, wheat grass

☐ Pituitary balance: use amino acids and homeopathic remedies

☐ Hypothalamus balance: amino acids and homeopathic remedies

Essential Fatty Acids

☐ Organic flaxseeds (ground) or oil

☐ Organic primrose and borage oil

☐ EPA: (eicosapentaenoic acid) (wild fish)

☐ DHA (docosahexaenoic acid) (wild fish)

Liver/Gallbladder/Kidney/Blood/ Colon Detox

☐ Gallbladder/Liver/Kidney Flush Kit

☐ Liver health: N-acetyl cysteine

☐ Bladder health: uva ursi

Mental Clarity

☐ GABA (amino acid)

☐ Ginkgo biloba (herb)

☐ Vinpocetine (derived from vincamine, an extract of the dwarf periwinkle plant, *Vinca minor*)

☐ DMAE (dimethyl amino ethanol)

☐ Phosphatidyl serine

☐ N-acetyl carnitine

Sleep

☐ GABA—Valerian-passionflower root combination

☐ Theanine

Now that we've discussed how you can nurture yourself by using food and supplements, please congratulate yourself. You have gained valuable nutritional knowledge and now can use many scientifically validated strategies to promote radiant health and hormone balance. In the next chapter, you'll learn the ins and outs of stress, along with stress-busting strategies for maximizing your strength in every area of your life.

Step 4 Action Plan

1. Please take the Mineral Self-Assessment Test, if you haven't done so already.
2. Take daily notes about how you feel on your hormone-balancing diet, so that you can track your progress. Be sure to note how different foods affect your mind and body.
3. Introduce new supplements into your diet, one at a time, and keep track of how they affect your physical and mental energy level.
4. Realize that sometimes it may be impossible to eat a hormone-healthful meal, such as when you're traveling or dining out. When this happens, reassure yourself that you're doing the best you can, and plan your next meal so that it's a healthful one.

Step 5

Stress and Hormone-Revitalization Strategies

Dr. Joanne is an internist who often consults with me on how to help her patients heal. This time she sought me out to help herself. Like many dedicated, compassionate doctors, Joanne works long and stressful hours, eats poorly, and has little time to enjoy herself. She reported feeling "stressed out to the max," so I gave her a hormone saliva test.

The results told an epic story of stress and hormone imbalance. While Dr. Joanne's estradiol measured nearly zero, her testosterone was low and her cortisol stayed low most of the day but zoomed upward at night. (High nighttime cortisol often manifests in people who cannot get going in the morning and have difficulty going to sleep at night.) She felt fatigued and weepy and ate sweets whenever she became stressed out. Dr. Joanne used coffee to keep her going and wine and chocolate to relax. "Sugar instead of sex," she told me.

Her low cortisol levels indicated that Dr. Joanne suffered from adrenal fatigue. Hence, we started by rebuilding her adrenal glands. She went on the detoxification diet, drank the revitalizing juice religiously, and used the Food Pyramid chart to make smart food choices. She even began to use my recipes (found in part 3). I taught her some deep breathing and meditation techniques to manage her stress. These gave her the power to relax her body and mind whenever she felt herself slipping into stress mode.

After a few months, her adrenal glands were back in healthy shape, and Dr. Joanne had so much energy that she no longer craved sugar or coffee to keep her going. What's more, her other hormone levels started to get back to normal, and so did her sex drive. Stressors in her life had become much more manageable, Dr. Joanne reported, and she found that taking more time to consciously relax and exercise helped to improve her moods.

Stress in Broad Strokes

As you know, and as Dr. Joanne could tell you, there are many types of stress, which can manifest in different forms of disease, such as breast cancer or depression. To convey how stress can influence a woman's physical and emotional history, I want to briefly mention how medicine has treated women's stress over the years and has often missed healing the source of stress, which happens to be hormonal imbalance.

Dr. Martin Charcot (1825–1893) was a highly esteemed and influential physician in nineteenth-century Europe. Practicing in the Paris hospital La Salpêtrière, Dr. Charcot's dubious specialty was hysteria. He diagnosed an average of ten hysterical women each day, effectively labeling them mentally ill outcasts. Compared to those dark ages of women's health, today we are in empowerment mode when it comes to treating stress.

Stress, as defined in the dictionary, means mental and physical tension or strain. When stress overwhelms the body and the mind, it sets numerous physical and emotional changes in motion. Stress can cause major personality transformations. You know you're stressed when you feel that your capability to meet responsibilities and challenges is overwhelmed by their magnitude. However, do keep in mind that you are not your stress.

I'm sure you'll agree that most of today's threats are psychological. After all, we often experience a full-blown stress response in everyday situations. You may already know from painful experience that a physical reaction to these events can wreak havoc on your mind/body health. Like many women, you may experience stress-related headaches, PMS, insomnia, digestive problems, or ulcers on an occasional or regular basis.

Stress may also make you feel tense, overwhelmed, enraged, depressed, hopeless, or exhausted. Other symptoms of stress include irritability, high blood pressure, headaches, weakening of the immune system, elevation of cholesterol levels, sleeplessness, migraine headaches, neck aches, diarrhea, dizziness, and loss of appetite. When stressors linger and continue to disrupt normal healthy functions, more serious illnesses may occur.

In fact, stress has been identified as a major cofactor in common illnesses and diseases such as depression, hypertension, heart disease, cancer, ulcers, stroke, and more. I assure you that you can free yourself from stress and illness. You can balance your hormones and enjoy good health.

In this chapter, you'll learn how to control stress so that you feel relaxed, strong, and capable. As I tell all my patients, it helps to breathe deeply while silently repeating to yourself the mantra, "I am not my stress. I am calm and capable."

Do you remember the discussion of stress and cortisol in chapter 2? You will learn much, much more about the cortisol-stress hookup in the following pages. By the end of this chapter, you'll also understand how stress impairs optimal brain function and memory and will learn stress management strategies that can revitalize your brain and the neurotransmitters that help keep your hormones in balance.

Given that twenty-first-century life is packed with stressors, like twenty-four-hour, seven-day work weeks, corporate downsizing, economic uncertainty, cyber-stress, and terrorist threats that elevate our blood pressure several times a day, it's safe to say that stress levels are at an all-time high. Robert Sapolsky, Ph.D., a Stanford University professor of neuroscience, has spent decades in the wild studying the stress response of baboons, our biological cousins. According to him, a convincing body of data supports the idea that stress levels increased markedly in the latter part of the twentieth century. Comparing 2000 with, say, 1950, "There is very solid data showing increasing rates of depression," says Dr. Sapolsky. "This data reflects, I believe, increasing amounts of psychological stress."

It's been estimated that 75 to 90 percent of all visits to primary-care physicians are for stress-related problems. While job stress is clearly the leading source of stress for adults, stress levels have also skyrocketed in children, teenagers, college students, and the elderly, for reasons that include the sustained use of computers; increased crime, violence, and other threats to personal safety; daily peer pressures that lead to substance abuse and other unhealthful habits; social isolation; and divorce.

In addition, the lack of close family members living nearby and the fragmented, impersonal nature of many communities have left scores of people feeling bereft of social support, which has been proven to foster stress in certain individuals.

We have stressors from our environment, which we can try to avoid or deny, but they still remain stressors. Then we have stressors that come from our emotional reactions to situations, events, our jobs, or relationships. These types of stressors can be eliminated as we learn to manage our emotions more calmly and carefully. We often need to just let the stress go. I assure you that you can do this. Here's an exercise that helps you release it, and I mean permanently. I call it the Bliss Exercise.

This self-liberating exercise teaches you how to still your mind and soothe your emotions, almost as effectively as if you are meditating. Here's how to begin:

1. Bring a chair outside where there are flowers, trees, and other beauties of nature. Sit with your feet flat on the ground. Take deep connected breaths by breathing in through your nose and out your mouth about ten times.

2. With your eyes wide open, look at a natural object, such as a flower, a tree, or a plant.

3. Feel the object's form and energy flow into your heart area. Never judge the object, think about it, or talk to it; just bring it into your heart space. See the form of an object and bring it into your heart, while taking deep connected breaths. Don't think about how to do it; just do it!

4. Now, speed up the process, and bring one form after another into your heart, taking no longer than two seconds for each.

5. Do this for ten minutes the first time. If a thought comes drifting into your mind, let it go and continue.

6. When you're finished, you'll notice that your mind is blissfully still. Enjoy!

If you do this every day, the positive effects are cumulative.

I'd like to share with you another technique, called the relaxation response, that helps you quickly produce a sense of calm even during a stressful situation at work or in public. (You can do this on the bus or the train.) If you're in an office environment, find an empty conference room to sit in or close your office door.

1. Find a quiet space to sit or lie down in comfort.

2. Choose a calming sound, word, phrase, or prayer. Repeat it silently or aloud.

3. Close your eyes and relax your muscles, progressing from your feet to your calves, thighs, abdomen, shoulders, head, and neck.

4. Breathe slowly and naturally, saying your phrase, sound, prayer, or word as you exhale.

5. Feel the resonance of the sound of your voice vibrate through your body. Never worry about how well you are relaxing. When distracting thoughts arise, simply notice them and then let them go, returning to the sound, the word, the phrase, or the prayer.

6. Start doing the relaxation response for ten minutes at a time. Continue to experience it for increasingly longer periods of time. It's that easy. Open your eyes and feel the calmness of your body and mind. Sit there for a minute before getting back on your feet. Dr. Benson and other researchers have confirmed that the relaxation response can be experienced while dancing, swimming, jogging, knitting, or doing yoga or qi gong.

Each of us has our own individual tolerance level for stress-related incidents. At one time or another, we've all reached our personal breaking points and lashed out in anger, frustration, or impatience because of outside influences that pushed our buttons and made us feel crazy. To learn more about how life events can stress an individual, the medical profession has invented various stress indexes. The Holmes-Rahe Stress Index is considered the gold standard for measuring stress.

The Holmes-Rahe Stress Index

Many years ago, Drs. Thomas H. Holmes and Richard H. Rahe at the University of Washington Medical School created an index of stressful events that has become a standard tool for health professionals to understand their patients' stressors and how to go about treating them. Hundreds of people of various ages and socioeconomic situations ranked the relative amount of adjustment that was required of them to meet a series of life events. Holmes and Rahe dubbed this "the social readjustment scale." The final numerical rating resulted from the average number of points these people assigned to the various life events, after being informed that marriage equaled fifty points.

According to Drs. Holmes and Rahe, any dramatic change that a person undergoes, whether it's perceived as welcome or unwelcome, causes stress, leaving us more vulnerable to disease.

For decades, mental health professionals have known that many of us create long-term stress and look for something to worry about because it feels like a comfortable shoe: very familiar. If the stress is short term, it can be managed without consequence. It is long-term chronic stress that causes the body to break down.

When you understand the degree to which you may be creating your own stress, it can feel daunting, depressing, or liberating. Why liberating? Because if you realize that you're creating your own stress, then you have the awesome power to nip stress in the bud.

Many people think they are just nervous and can never change. It's a fact that stress first affects parts of the body that are closely related to the nervous system, such as the digestive and the intestinal systems. This clearly indicates that chronic indigestion or colitis may be totally related to stressors, either emotional or environmental. Before you assess your adrenal stress and learn some stress-relieving tools, let's consider hidden stresses that are often overlooked by the general public and the medical community.

Hidden Health Stressors

In my practice, I help patients to heal their body, mind, and spirit, naturally through the NeuroPhysical Reprogramming (NPR) process. Time and again, I find that the cause of disease often originates in one or more of these three areas: dental health, the mind/body connection, and genetics. It's essential to examine these aspects of your health to discover the source of your conditions.

From twenty years' experience, I know that if you locate and heal the cause, you can permanently heal the disease. Yes, any disease. For example, because every organ, system, gland, vertebra, and acupuncture meridian is related to your teeth, dental health critically influences wellness. Unlike most internists, when I see a patient, I always review the health of the individual's teeth, especially in people who have root canals, fillings, and crowns. Most of the substances that dentists put inside your teeth are toxic.

Before you get dental treatment, you can have a blood test done that will indicate biocompatible substances for your body. Electrodermal screening, kinesiology, or the NPR technique that I invented may also work well for biocompatibility testing. I suggest that you visit a biological dentist in your area who specializes in this field of holistic health. A biological dentist has been trained in using nontoxic, biocompatible substances, rather than mercury amalgam fillings, and uses special methods to keep you from ingesting the toxic substances that are being removed. See the dental chart on page 206 and see the Resource Guide for information on finding a biological dentist.

I want to note a few other insidious, obscure stressors that are often overlooked. As I mentioned in chapter 3, the agricultural industry's prodigious use of prescription drugs, growth hormones, and antibiotics on poultry, cattle, and swine farms has caused these substances to reach toxic levels in our water supply. The drugs then silently stress our bodies by taxing our immune systems and lowering our resistance to viruses, bacteria, and various diseases.

The American public's dependence on antibiotics, antidepressants, conventional and natural hormones, cholesterol-lowering drugs, and so on, has led to drugs and drug metabolites finding their way into our water supply each year. No one knows the long-term health consequences of ingesting these drugs and drug-breakdown products or how they may affect our moods, emotions, or mental health.

I think of these drugs as toxic tiles in the complex mosaic of manmade, or iatrogenic, disease—an epidemic that characterizes twenty-first-century U.S. life. We need to take action and prevent stress causing disease whenever we can. If you remained unconvinced by my suggestions to get a water filter and a purifier, perhaps you'll reconsider now. I assure you that it will make a valuable difference in your immune system's ability to combat viruses, bacteria, and toxins. As you become aware, rather than paranoid, you can use this information to make wiser lifestyle choices that contribute to a sexier, more vital new you.

Continuing with livestock-related stressors, it's imperative that you understand the health risks related to eating beef. Mad cow disease, also known as BSE, is a real, present, and lethal illness endangering meat eaters around the world. Here's the spin: the U.S. Department of Agriculture claims that BSE is found only in the brain and the nervous system of the animal, and that eating other parts of a diseased cow is safe if the brain and the nervous system are removed.

The truth is that if the cow is infected, every part of the cow has BSE. Therefore, you can get mad cow disease from eating any part of the animal. How do I know this is the truth? Because if a virus is in the brain, and the blood goes to the brain and circulates throughout the organism, it's possible that the virus can spread throughout the body, just as cancer initially located in one organ can spread throughout the body. If there is a possible cure for BSE, it lies in the realm of homeopathy—drugs generally control the disease, but do not cure it.

Many people get treated for allergies, which are certainly stressors, yet these may not be the root cause of certain health problems. If you have an illness, the first assessment should be determining the health of your immune system. An overburdened and underpowered immune system may be the root cause of any allergy, such as one to weeds, grasses, wheat, trees, and so forth. If you haven't already taken the Biological Age Assessment Quiz in chapter 3, please do so, for it will help you evaluate your immunity. You'll find nutritional recommendations for specific conditions in chapter 4, as well as homeopathic remedies in chapter 7.

The Cortisol-Stress Connection

Cortisol is the primary stress hormone, and the cortisol-stress connection hugely influences your hormones, your memory, and your moods.

Cortisol production is essentially triggered by the pituitary hormone ACTH (adrenocorticotropin hormone). During a stressful moment, the pituitary receives red alerts from the hypothalamus in the form of the hormone CRH, or corticotropin-releasing hormone, to release ACTH. This ACTH secretion instructs the adrenal glands to increase cortisol production and secretion. Almost immediately after a stressful event, ACTH and CRH flood the bloodstream, causing an immediate spike in cortisol levels.

When cortisol is present in excess amounts, a negative feedback system operates on the pituitary gland and the hypothalamus. The hypothalamus commands these areas to restrict the output of ACTH and CRH, in order to reduce cortisol secretion when adequate levels are present.

While this happens, other body tissues downsize their use of glucose as fuel. Cortisol secretion also leads to the release of fatty acids, an energy source from fat cells, for use by the muscles. Your body relies on an elaborate hormonal feedback system to control cortisol secretion and regulate the amount of cortisol in the bloodstream. A constant conversation is going on between your stress and pituitary hormones, your brain, your memory, and your blood. Cortisol irregularities, however, can interrupt that conversation and can damage your endocrine glands. This can make you gain weight and can stress your brain and body in subtle, yet profound, ways.

For example, cortisol release during the stress response can cause an immediate short-term memory deficit. Perhaps you've had an accident or a stressful experience that you can remember only in fragments. Dr. Sapolsky and others have shown that cortisol secretion decreases blood sugar utilization by the brain's chief memory center, the hippocampus.

Low blood sugar in the hippocampus makes the brain deficient in the material that chemically records memories. Sustained cortisol release also jams neurotransmitter functions, meaning that even if a joyous or relaxing memory has been recorded in the past, your brain cannot access it now.

Cortisol-induced communication breakdown makes it hard for brain cells to converse with each other. Thoughts get confused, and the thinker feels mentally paralyzed for a moment. Overproduction of cortisol also thrashes brain cells by causing excessive amounts of calcium to invade them, producing the dreaded free radicals that you read about in chapter 4.

The brain derives most of its energy from glucose, so it's crucial that you maintain adequate blood levels. If you fast, cortisol output increases, and this activates catabolism, or the breakdown of protein into basic amino acids and their conversion into glucose to feed the brain. Clockwork production of adrenal glucocorticoids is essential for optimal health. In normal individuals, the breakdown of tissues by glucocorticoids is followed by the building up of tissues by androgens (male hormones).

As we grow older, a surplus of catabolic hormones over anabolic hormones develops. This is one reason why our body tissues age and we lose our youthful ability to repair damaged tissues. The same thing occurs under chronic, excessive stress, which contributes to premature aging.

Hidden Thyroid, Parathyroid, and Adrenal Stressors

There is a popular myth that the thyroid gland can never be healed. Physicians routinely inform patients that once they start taking a thyroid medication, which is, of course, hormone replacement, they must continue taking it for the rest of their life. Conventional medicine teaches physicians how to administer thyroid medications, instead of how to heal thyroid imbalances holistically without drugs. The fact is, certain homeopathic protocols, simple foods, and herbal remedies can bring thyroid function back to health.

As a matter of fact, I healed my own thyroid, which was weakened by exposure to nuclear radiation that drifted from the Chernobyl nuclear reactor in the former Soviet Union and into Germany, where I studied in the mid-1980s. I healed it with thrice-weekly saunas and by taking a daily dose of the vitamin niacin and homeopathic remedies specifically designed to remove nuclear radiation from the body. I have helped men and women on long-term (twenty-five years) thyroid treatment heal their thyroids and stop using prescription medications. The immune system can be strengthened, and the part of the thyroid that is left can be returned to a normal level of functioning, without prescription medicines. With most of my patients, it took six months to one year to get their thyroids working normally.

Because the thyroid is so important to your hormones and overall health, I will give you the fundamentals of the program that I prescribe to my patients to heal this gland. Naturally, the dosages will vary according to the individual. However, along with detoxification of medications, I detox the thyroid gland by working with the emotions of the thyroid (confusion and paranoia) and using customized nutrition and homeopathy. I also recommend eating foods that are known to heal the thyroid. It's vital to eliminate foods that harm the adrenal and the thyroid glands, such as caffeine and sugar. While caffeine depletes the adrenal glands and thyroid, sugar exhausts the pancreas, the spleen, and the adrenals.

People with adrenal problems often have their thyroid function evaluated through blood tests that fail to accurately measure thyroid health. Therefore, they may never find out the true condition of their thyroid, which may be super-stressed. The thyroid and the adrenal glands belong to the same element, which is Fire, according to Traditional Chinese Medicine's Five Element Theory.

If you have adrenal problems, I recommend a Five Element Hormone Saliva Test. This measures hormone levels throughout the day, including at 10:00 P.M., which is the thyroid time in traditional Chinese medicine. You may want to refresh your memory of the Five Element Theory and its corresponding organs and times of day by reviewing the chart found at the end of chapter 2.

Whenever hypo- or hyperthyroid function problems exist, so do adrenal gland weaknesses. In addition, other hidden causes of some thyroid problems can include a dysfunctional pituitary and possibly the hypothalamus. *Because the thyroid and the adrenal glands work in tandem, it's vital that they be treated simultaneously.* You can learn more about this on my Web site (see the Resource Guide). Look for an article about NeuroEmotional Remedies.

Adrenal Stress Indicators

Adrenal stress comes from excessive cortisol release that is experienced during the stress response. I gauge adrenal stress with the help of hormone saliva tests. Let's look at the different indicators and phases of this condition.

> *Phase 1, Adrenal adaptation*: Symptoms include digestive problems, inability to calm down, increased serum cholesterol, severe weight gain or loss, menstrual problems, sleep disturbances, diarrhea, decrease in sex drive

Phase 2, Adrenal maladaption: Symptoms include chronic fatigue syndrome, loss of libido, impotence, bloating and fluid retention, constipation, male or female hair loss, bone loss, increased urination, low back or sciatica pain

Phase 3, Adrenal exhaustion: Symptoms include fibromyalgia; chronic, nonspecific pain; heart arrhythmia; severe constipation; panic attacks or anxiety; bile reflux and digestive problems; depression and mental frustration; memory loss and inability to think; sensitivity to smells, light, or sound; difficulty breathing; inflammation; joint pain

Phase 4, Blood sugar events: Symptoms include a possible hypoglycemic condition if one or two cortisol levels are elevated. Genetic predisposition for diabetes is possible if two or more cortisol levels are elevated for an extended time. The higher the cortisol level, the more likely are blood sugar problems and diabetes.

Now you've got a clear picture of what your brain and your body go through when you're under adrenal stress, as well as what hidden stressors can do to your health. Take the following Adrenal Stress Self-Assessment Test to get an idea of how stress may be affecting your hormones.

Adrenal Stress Self-Assessment Test

Please check all that apply to you.

Adrenal Deficiency
- ☐ fatigue
- ☐ craving for sugar
- ☐ allergies
- ☐ chemical sensitivity
- ☐ stress
- ☐ heart palpitations
- ☐ arthritis
- ☐ aches and pains
- ☐ irritability
- ☐ decreased concentration
- ☐ low body temperature

Adrenal Excess
- ☐ bone loss
- ☐ fatigue
- ☐ weight gain, primarily around waist
- ☐ sleep disturbance, insomnia
- ☐ elevated triglycerides
- ☐ breast cancer
- ☐ irritability, anxiety, nervousness
- ☐ depression
- ☐ headaches

☐ low libido

☐ hair loss

☐ increased facial hair (women)

☐ increased body hair (women)

☐ acne

☐ memory lapses

Now total the boxes checked in either column.

If you have two boxes checked in either column and symptoms are persistent for two months or more, saliva testing is indicated and perhaps a visit to one of my affiliates (see the Resource Guide). You will also definitely want to practice some of the stress-management strategies in this chapter and check out remedies in chapter 7's homeopathy chart.

Neurotransmitters and Stress

As you learned in chapter 2, neurotransmitters are chemicals that relay signals between nerve cells. Neurotransmitters hugely influence your emotional stability, drive and motivation, ability to focus, mental alertness, memory making and retrieval, positive feelings for yourself and others, calmness in the face of challenges, digestion, and sleep.

Any form of chronic stress can greatly affect neurotransmitter levels. So can genetics, environment, diet, exercise, medications, chemical exposure, and substance abuse. If the body is low in certain amino acids, then neurotransmitter depletion or imbalance can occur; this can be a major source of body/mind stress.

Five neurotransmitters (serotonin, catecholamine, dopamine, epinephrine, and norepinephrine) and the amino acid neurotransmitter called GABA are required for proper brain function; suboptimal or deficient levels can cause serious health problems. The main neurotransmitters that are affected by stress are the "feel good" or excitatory neurotransmitters and the inhibitory neurotransmitters.

Excitatory neurotransmitters include endorphins, the body's natural opioids or painkillers. These are mood-elevating and can bring on euphoria. Researchers have found low levels of endorphins in women suffering from PMS. While exercise promotes endorphin release, so can creative visualization of someone or something you love, laughing, listening to music, and enjoying other pleasurable activities. Perhaps the most satisfying endorphin release is sexual arousal and, of course, orgasm.

Norepinephrine, an antidepressant that also makes you feel energized and keeps the appetite in check, also flows during times of sexual arousal. Dopamine promotes feelings of bliss and pleasure. Ahhh. It plays a big role in addiction, appetite control, and mental focus. It also helps to regulate motor control and body movements.

The excitatory neurotransmitter glutamate is essential for balanced brain chemistry and brain health. Research has linked glutamate imbalance to bipolar disorder and attention deficit hyperactivity disorder (ADHD). Acetylcholine helps in the release of human growth hormone, while supporting alertness, memory, and appetite control. This fantastic substance also promotes sexual arousal and romantic performance—yet another reason why you want your diet to provide you with all of the essential amino acids.

Rounding out the excitatory neurotransmitters, phenylethylamine (PEA) delights your body with blissful feelings and sensations. It is heavily involved in feelings of infatuation. . . . No wonder high levels of PEA are found in chocolate! Beta-phenylethylamine (PEA) is an amine neurotransmitter derived from the amino acid phenylalanine. Studies of PEA have found that it promotes energy and elevates mood. PEA also functions as a synaptic neuromodulator inhibiting the reuptake of dopamine and norepinephrine. PEA is lipid soluble and readily crosses the blood-brain barrier. Studies have shown that patients with depression and those with ADD/ADHD have decreased PEA levels while levels are increased in schizophrenic and psychopathic subjects. It has also been implicated in migraines and the antidepressant effects of exercise.

As for inhibitory neurotransmitters, enkephalins restrict pain transmission and reduce cravings and depression. GABA, or gamma-aminobutyric acid, is found throughout the central nervous system. An antistress, antianxiety, anti-panic, and anti-pain substance, GABA helps you to feel calm and maintain control and focus.

Serotonin prevents agitated depression and worrying; it also promotes sleep and improves self-esteem. Serotonin helps to diminish craving as well. This is the neurotransmitter that presumably most of us are deficient in. Serotonin is the same substance that Prozac, one of the most popular antidepressants, helps to redistribute in the brain.

Known as the rest-and-recuperation or antiaging hormone, melatonin regulates the body's internal clock and assists in helping you fall asleep. Oxytocin, which is stimulated by dopamine, promotes sexual arousal, feelings of emotional attachment, and the desire to cuddle.

If you exercise; get at least eight hours of sleep a night; avoid caffeine, alcohol, and drugs; and follow the dietary recommendations in chapter 4, this will help you to manage stress and maintain a healthy neurotransmitter balance. So will practicing the relaxation exercises and hormone-balancing meditation described at the end of this chapter.

Soothing Stress with Nutritional Supplements

I'm not big on prescribing lots of vitamins, but I often recommend certain nutrients to help with stressful times in my patients' lives. The following suggestions should be tried out one supplement at a time. I recommend that you take these for no longer than one month because your body changes very quickly and your needs for nutrients also change. The nutrients and dosages on this list have helped my patients to balance their internalized stress. You'll find these supplements in the health food store and some supermarkets. I'm sure that one or more of them will help you feel calmer, stronger, and sexier.

Take phosphatidyl choline if you have low cortisol levels; follow label instructions.

Take phosphatidyl serine if you have high cortisol levels; follow label instructions.

The B-complex vitamins can help to reduce damage to the immune system; take vitamin B-complex, 100 mg daily.

Take magnesium citrate or glycinate, 1,000 mg per day. (Best taken in the evening.)

L-tyrosine (amino acid), 500 mg in the morning, 500 mg at bedtime, helps to reduce the effects of stress on the body.

Take calcium orotate, 1,500 mg per day.

Vitamin C with bioflavonoids and rutin, 3,000–10,000 mg per day, is essential for adrenal gland function (stress depletes the adrenal gland hormones).

Kelp, 5 tablets per day, is a balanced vitamin/mineral preparation and is also good for hypothyroid conditions.

L-lysine, plus vitamin C and zinc gluconate, taken as directed on the label, will help cold sores because it helps neutralize stress (cold sores may be caused by herpes, which is aggravated by stress). Stress causes vitamin depletion, and vitamin C is essential for the entire body. It helps to rebuild the body.

A multivitamin and mineral complex containing vitamin A, 25,000 IU daily, should be taken in divided doses.

Potassium, 99 mg daily, is needed for adrenal gland function.

Proteolytic enzymes, between meals, destroy free radicals released by stress.

Vitamin E mixed tocopherols, at least 400 IU daily, helps the immune system.

Zinc, 50 mg daily, helps the immune system.

A few herbs that are effective for relieving chronic stress include chamomile, hops, lavender flowers, lemon balm, lotus plumule, passionflower, pau d'arco, Saint-John's wort, and valerian root. These can be used to alleviate short-term stress. Remember, avoid becoming dependent on any substance.

Certain homeopathic remedies for stress take into account individual personality characteristics, which will help you make a more permanent shift in how you internalize and deal with stress. You will find these in chapter 7.

Stress-Management Tool Kit

1. Stress-balancing meditation. This meditation fosters health, relaxation, and hormone balance. It involves visualizing the amygdala, a part of the brain that's intimately involved in processing emotions, especially fear. I created this meditation based on my understanding of how women's adrenal glands, often starting in the

teenage years, become exhausted from habitually slipping into the stress response whenever they've consumed too much caffeine or are anxious, afraid, or just trying to meet a deadline or care for a family member.

Treating hormonal imbalance at the source is one of my main endeavors as a healer. This meditation is a powerful tool in your healing arsenal, mainly because it calms the adrenal glands by inducing a deep relaxation response. Moreover, when you relax the adrenal glands, this reduces the severity of PMS or menopausal symptoms. In fact, my patients report that practicing this meditation will even lessen symptoms such as anxiety, breast tenderness, and hot flashes.

Another reason why it's good for you to practice this meditation is that people tend to react to stressors the way they learned to during childhood. This meditation can change your old way of handling stress into a new mastery over stress. Are you ready to try it? Good, here's how.

Find a comfortable space. Place your feet flat on the floor and your arms on your legs, with palms up toward the sky.

Inhale slowly through your nose. Feel and imagine the breath going all the way up to the third eye space between your eyes, then exhale down your spine to your coccyx bone. Now, immediately inhale again but this time from your coccyx bone: visualize and feel your breath going around your genitals to the front of your body and up and back to the third eye. You are making a circle. Continue breathing like this, slowly connecting the breaths, for about five minutes until it becomes natural.

While breathing deep connected breaths, turn your closed eyes gently toward the third eye area. Breathe and gently gaze toward the place between your eyebrows for another three minutes.

After three minutes, breathe normally but keep your gaze up toward your third eye area. Immediately, place the tip of your tongue on the roof of your mouth with your mouth closed.

Now visualize that a feather is inside your brain, gently tickling your amygdala.

Very gently tickle that area and feel the feather, ever so slightly. Continue tickling the amygdala for approximately four minutes. See it with your mind's eye, and you'll feel your body and mind relax and then feel rejuvenated. The next step is to keep your awareness on the amygdala, the hypothalamus, and the pituitary while you hold your tongue on the roof of your mouth. Keep tickling with the feather and breathing. Now imagine your hypothalamus and pituitary as orchestra leaders communicating through music with your ovaries, thyroid, and adrenals, sending musical frequencies that support production of proper amounts of hormones and healthy endocrine function. You may play calming classical music during this exercise.

After approximately fifteen to twenty minutes, you'll feel relaxed, yet aware and balanced. This exercise can be done daily, for as long as you like.

2. Biofeedback for stress management. For many years, I've used professional biofeedback devices and battery-operated, hand-held biofeedback units to track the effect of stress on the body and to help my patients learn how to manage their stress by inducing the relaxation response. All of these biofeedback tools track your heart rhythms in real time, to illustrate your immediate emotional and physical state.

There are even biofeedback computer programs with fingertip sensors that track your heart rhythms and plug into your computer so that you can practice relaxing in the middle of your workday. PC-based computer biofeedback programs contain exercises that quickly teach you how to lower your heart rate, which in turn helps to reduce blood pressure and stress hormones, while increasing antiaging hormones. (A graph of spiky, erratic lines shows that you're angry or stressed, while flowing ones signify serenity or happiness.) There are also wristwatch-sized, computerized heart rhythm monitors that help you shift into the relaxation response. See the Resource Guide for facts on biofeedback devices and appendix B for information on electromagnetic energy.

3. Exercise, your body's best friend. One major reason why the National Institutes of Health (NIH) calls exercise "the most effective antiaging pill ever discovered" is its effect on hormones. Along with inducing the self-healing relaxation response, physical exercise raises levels of norepinephrine, a key hormone for maintaining a positive mood. Norepinephrine also functions as a neurotransmitter that helps to create new memories; it's primarily

responsible for moving them from short-term to long-term storage. To reap the full stress-management benefits of exercise, you must exercise at least four days per week.

Hands down, exercise beats HRT for keeping your bones strong. Besides reducing stress, exercise wins out over HRT for helping bone density. Let's compare the two.

First, HRT induces unwanted weight gain, while exercise burns calories by speeding up the metabolism, promoting a low body weight. In chapters 1 and 2, we reviewed statistics proving that HRT puts you at risk of getting breast cancer, while exercise *reduces* this risk. When it comes to cost, exercise also has HRT beat: you have no physician visits or pharmaceutical agents to purchase.

Now let's consider your mental health for a moment. People using HRT have increased risks of getting Alzheimer's and dementia, yet exercise may lower this risk. Exercising outdoors has another benefit: sunshine causes the body to produce vitamin D. Volumes of research prove that vitamin D increases bone density, by stimulating more calcium absorption in the gut and depositing more calcium into the bone matrix. HRT does not do this.

I vary my exercise routine, to keep myself interested and amused. With my schedule, I try to exercise in the privacy of my home, except for Bikram yoga classes, which I enjoy at least three times per week. I do Pilates four to five evenings per week at home and in the morning use my exercise ball and light weights and work out with various aerobic VHS tapes. (Working out with light weights is important for all women as a means to strengthen bone and manage weight. A famous Tufts University research study that compared women who followed identical diet plans found that the strength-training group lost 44 percent more fat than did the diet-only group. (See the Resource Guide for recommended reading on strength training.)

I also enjoy jumping on my little trampoline and using my inversion bed. Most of this equipment is inexpensive, especially when you compare it to medical bills that you may spare yourself from! Moreover, on weekends I enjoy hiking or power walking and am starting to learn qi gong. Years of counseling patients has taught me that most people dread exercising because they don't like it. If you engage in different kinds of exercise, though, you'll surely find workouts that make you feel great and keep your mind amused.

While Pilates, qi gong, yoga, light weight lifting, jogging, walking, swimming, and cycling are all recommended forms of exercise, one type of exercise happens to promote bone health more than others do. It's called vibratory motion, says Dennis Lobstein, Ph.D., an exercise psychobiologist based in Miami, Florida, and the coauthor of the sports training guide *Consistent Winning*.

Vibratory motion torques the bone and allows more electrical current (scientists call this the piezoelectric effect) to flow around the bone, which in turn promotes increased levels of calcium deposited inside. All forms of dance are very effective for building bone, and so is qi gong or judo, says Dr. Lobstein, who has practiced martial arts for the last thirty years and is a medical qi gong practitioner. Training with resistance weights has also proved to promote stress management and bone-building power, while conferring extraordinary fat-fighting and metabolism-boosting benefits.

Realize that even moderate exercises have dramatic effects on bone density. You can combine easy, low-resistance bone exercises with your cardiovascular workout to save time. Dr. Lobstein recommends that you engage in a variety of exercises at least three, but not more than five, times per week. You can overdose if you exercise five days in a row, which will increase the risk of illness, injury, and burnout, as it doesn't allow your body to recover and become stronger.

Moreover, rest periods of two full days in a row have an important function in the recovery process. Overtraining actually causes bone atrophy, which is opposite from the effect that you want to achieve. Whether you are power walking, jumping, jogging, cycling, or swimming, you can enhance your workout by following these suggestions.

- Cardiovascular workout: use ankle and/or wrist weights and wear them during your workout. Start with low half-pound weights and build up to more. You can speed up and slow down to get used to the weights. Wilderness hiking with this technique is great, but use the buddy system until you know your limits.

- Jumping up and down on a trampoline is fun, too.
- Jumping rope and skipping with ankle and/or wrist weights is fun and effective.
- I prefer to do my power walking on the beach or in the mountains.
- The same principles with weights can be applied to cycling; vary your hills or terrain.
- With swimming, you can wear waterproof weights and move slowly through the water, using the water as resistance. Start in the shallow end and do some power walking in the water. Move deeper for more challenge, swimming and treading water at liberty.

Power stretching is important, because it prevents injury. You can power stretch with weights, but be careful and move slowly for starters. Besides stimulating more bone density, stretching will help your connective tissue. Be sure to stretch before and after your workout. Stretching makes the connective tissue more pliable, laying down collagen and elastin (the elastic proteins in connective tissue) along the lines of force that you create with your movements.

People who never stretch or exercise lay down their connective tissue at random; this makes it weaker and more prone to injury, says Dr. Lobstein. Quick, forceful, jerky movements, which you're likely to make while wearing weights, put the connective tissue at more risk of injury. Good areas to stretch include hamstrings, legs, ankles, lower back, torso, arms, and neck.

Yoga is terrific for stretching; take it slow until you're confident of your flexibility. Here's a good index of your level of flexibility: can you bend over and touch your head to your knees, without bending your knees, and grab your ankles at the same time? If this is challenging, you have a worthwhile goal to work toward.

If you're just starting to exercise and stretch, take yoga or Pilates classes. If you have the time and the money, you could also visit a local exercise physiologist, a personal trainer, or an athletic trainer to help you with specific movements.

4. Guided imagery for stress relief. One of the easiest ways to manage stress is to practice guided imagery. This involves visualizing positive

situations and beautiful scenes; it has been shown in various studies to improve immune functioning and create healthier outcomes in cancer and heart patients. For instance, visualizing a loved one or even a favorite pet has been found to lower blood pressure and induce the relaxation response, which stimulates the release of endorphins, the body's natural painkillers. Books and tapes on guided imagery can be found in most libraries and bookstores.

5. Sound healing. Have you ever wondered why certain songs, nature sounds, or types of music make you feel ecstatic, soothed, or transported? Scientific research confirms that low-frequency sounds and vibrations, drumming, and various musical compositions can promote beneficial physiological and mental conditions without any negative side effects.

   Certain sounds can reduce stress, elevate mood, ease muscle tension, lower blood pressure, and increase immune system function. Many rhythms have also been found to shift brain waves from frantic beta into calm theta, a state where relaxation and creative thinking are possible. Why does sound exert such power over our minds and bodies? We are rhythmical beings whose hearts and minds are strongly influenced by external rhythms in the environment. In my practice, I've given my patients music therapy tools for over two decades to help them manage stress and induce the relaxation response.

   While a normal adult heart at rest pulses 60 to 100 beats per minute, the scientific law of rhythm entertainment describes how faster-paced environmental sounds stimulate the heart to synchronize with upbeat tempos. A pneumatic jackhammer, for instance, forces your heart rate to speed up in a race to entrain, or match, its fast pace. The jackhammer's speedy pace raises blood pressure, while stress hormones run riot. Breathing becomes shallow and irregular, and other organs and body systems fall out of their normal rhythms.

   An effective way to manage stress is by listening to slow classical acoustic music. Research using heart rate variability monitors at the Center for Neuroacoustic Research in Encinitas, California, and elsewhere confirms that listening to music that cycles at 60 beats per minute or less, such as Bach, reduces the heart rate and promotes effective stress management. (Tuning in to gently paced baroque, contemporary music, or nature sounds, such as ocean waves or crickets, can also provide identical stress-busting benefits.)

6. Self-massage and massage. Some of the documented benefits of self-massage and massage by certified therapists include increased blood flow, reduction of blood pressure and heart rate, endorphin and other excitatory neurotransmitter release, increased lymphatic drainage, and a rise in immune system functioning. You can use your own hands to massage your face, temples, neck, and hands. Health food stores also sell self-massage tools that are made of wood or are battery-operated.

   If you have the money and the time, booking a massage with a certified massage therapist can be remarkably helpful in managing your stress. Massage centers in shopping malls, airports, and health food stores also offer people on the go a chance to experience the benefits of healing touch.

Stress Tips I Give to My Patients

The following tips can help you handle difficult situations:

- Avoid caffeine, smoking, alcohol, and drugs. While drugs and alcohol may offer temporary relief from stress, they will never eliminate the source of it. Indeed, you may develop a dependency on drugs or alcohol that could trigger health problems, financial difficulties, and emotional turmoil, which further compound your stress.
- The detoxification diet and revitalization juice recipe in chapter 3 are basic stress-management tools.
- Exercise four times a week to stay calm, strong, and energized.
- Get proper rest each night to ensure optimal health.
- Do the hormone-balancing meditation every day.
- Try to get at least eight hours of sleep each night, if possible. The less rested you are, the weaker your immune system is. You'll also feel more stressed, and your chances of becoming ill are elevated because your immune system is strained.
- Deep breathing can help you shake off stress and can be done anywhere. Simply take a deep, slow, six-second inhalation when you're tense. Exhale for six seconds.

- Take a day off to avoid burning yourself out as Dr. Joanne did. This is what weekends are for.
- Take a drive, go to the beach, work in the yard, or read a book.
- Hobbies are great stress busters. Take the time to create, cook, or otherwise enjoy something for a few minutes or more each day.
- Never feel guilty about spending time and money doing something for yourself. Your health is worth it.
- Last, but not least, don't take life so seriously! Learn to laugh.

After you try all of the self-empowering, self-assessing, and self-healing tools in this chapter, I know that you'll feel a tremendous shift in your stress levels and your ability to cultivate calm and peace in the midst of challenging circumstances. Now you're ready to focus on healing and balancing your emotions, which is the subject of the next chapter.

Step 5 Action Plan

1. First take the Adrenal Stress Self-Assessment Test.
2. Get destressed by doing these workouts: Bikram yoga, hatha yoga, ashtanga yoga, or Pilates.
3. On your work breaks, close your eyes and breathe deeply. Take twenty-five diaphragmatic deep connected breaths, breathing in through your mouth all the way up to your third eye and out your nose.
4. Enjoy two good belly laughs per day.
5. Write up a list of nutrients that will be helpful, according to the results of the self-assessment tests, and determine how to get more of these into your daily diet.
6. Try a meditation today and see how relaxed you feel afterward.

Step 6

Emotional-Management Techniques for Inner Revitalization

Dorothy is thirty-eight years old. She has focused on her physical health for nearly a decade. One of the most dedicated people I've ever known, Dorothy expresses this dedication through body building, taking nutritional supplements, and engaging in frequent aerobic exercise. Dorothy came to me because she felt devastated by severe PMS, with constant migraines, depression, confusion, and uncontrollable rage.

Dorothy described herself as being on an emotional roller coaster and said that she often felt like she was losing control of her life. She said she could hardly get anything else done after her daily workout, due to fatigue and lack of focus.

Feeling a sense of urgency, I rushed the testing and worked quickly to help her before she sank deeper into despair. Her saliva test results indicated that four cortisol levels were low and two were very high, indicating a possible blood sugar disorder. I questioned her about her eating habits and body-building supplements. Dorothy's diet consisted mainly of animal protein, carbohydrates, whey, egg, and soy protein powders. This nutritionally unbalanced diet served her body poorly. Dorothy's endocrine and other systems were weakened from her deficiencies in fruits, vegetables, and whole grains. Even worse, for years she had consumed sugar-laden supplements, protein bars, and drinks to gain muscle mass.

After compiling information from testing and taking a case history about her life and childhood, I recommended a complete program that included emotional release work to help resolve her childhood and adult emotional-abuse issues. Dorothy was quite relieved to hear this and immediately took the Neuro-Emotional Self-Assessment Test at the end of this chapter. It was obvious from the test results that she needed to do some emotional work. She had checked ten major emotions that she felt at least 35 percent of the time each week. That's a lot of time to spend resisting your feelings and your family, and it took a heavy toll on her mind. It was easy to see why she had difficulty getting things done.

Dorothy and I had a compassionate "power talk" about her pressing emotional and physical problems. This resulted in our deciding to conduct two NeuroPhysical Reprogramming sessions per week for one month. NeuroPhysical Reprogramming (NPR) is a technique that I invented that pinpoints the cause of any life condition, determines its location in your body, and then allows you to permanently release it.

NPR incorporates an advanced form of muscle testing to determine the source of a condition and a method to locate and release resisted emotions, belief systems, and self-images that are stored in the body, creating abnormal energy flow and disease. These self-images become lodged in our bodies during childhood experiences. They are literally imprinted in our emotional and physical memories, living on in our unconscious, yet continually influencing our conscious life. Certain experiences trigger these emotions, belief systems, and self-images, which in turn trigger overwhelming and often negative emotions.

I also put Dorothy on the diet and nutritional programs described in chapters 3 and 4. By the time she finished the emotional release sessions, four weeks later, I must say, I hardly recognized her. She had liberated and fortified her mind and body. She said that she had never felt more normal or emotionally balanced. Dorothy continued with her new attitude and lifestyle. She enjoyed all the new positive reactions she received from her friends and family and found it easier to manage the stressors in her life.

Understanding Emotional Dependency

Our emotions can be hugely helpful passports, or else roadblocks, along the journey of life. Emotions are compounded of complex chemicals, beliefs, and events that allow us to experience happiness, joy, love, and, of course, sadness, anger, and fear. For decades, women have been misdiagnosed and mistreated by physicians who have told them that their uteruses or their minds were the cause of their emotional upset.

Even though it's old news, I'm still astonished that emotional issues have been labeled "hysteria" and then again relabeled "just hormones." What many health professionals are now embracing is how emotions can trigger emotional symptoms and hormonal imbalances.

One reason why emotions continue to be poorly understood by many physicians and healers is the way disease is conceptualized and treated in the West. There are two main models for treating disease. The first is the biochemical theory, and the second is the holistic or energetic approach. Herein lies the problem: biochemists view the human body as a chemical chain reaction, triggered by enzymes. How emotions fit into this model is a highly controversial and still emerging science.

Alternatively, in the holistic model of health, we're influenced by our environment, meditation, body work, supplements, and diet— not just by our enzymes. The only problem that I see with this holistic model is that we can become too dependent on it and cease to be aware of the emotional content of our lives. The fact is, you can become dependent on things that are widely perceived as healthful, such as love, exercise, meditation, nutritional supplements, and so forth.

In my view, the only way to avoid dependency is by consistently exploring, detecting, and feeling the emotional content of our lives. We must clearly see and feel how our emotions work, instead of being worked over by our emotions and numbing them through dependencies on various substances and activities. I'm happy to say that this chapter will give you some powerful tools to help you realize, and embody, your own emotional understanding and healing.

You Can Heal Your Emotions

Toward that end, let's first examine the emotional underpinnings of illness. Doing this will help to illuminate how your emotions can literally cause hormonal and other woes. Copious research indicates that many emotional problems lie deeply buried in our subconscious. Although we may courageously commit to a course of psychotherapy or psychiatry to understand the mystery of our personalities, we often never uncover the fundamental meaning of these mysteries.

Many of the talk therapies are designed to help you go back in your life, find the origin of your problems, and then talk them out. Unfortunately, this can be a long and unrewarding process for many people. Please understand that I don't condemn these therapies. I'm merely pointing out that they often fail to help many people resolve their emotional problems. Some of my patients have told me that talk therapy made them feel worse after they revisited their past traumas, and it kept them stuck in the same emotional confusion for years. If you rehash traumas every week for a year, you may never release them. Rather, you often keep them alive and kicking.

In Dorothy's case, the NPR protocol allowed her to bypass her conscious mind to reveal the underlying causes of her overwhelming emotions and chronic illnesses. Dorothy suffered from frequent candida albicans infections, viruses, flu, and gallstones, which she detoxed with the gallbladder/liver/kidney cleanse. It took a month and a half to completely detox her gallbladder and strengthen her immune system.

Since one of my main goals is to empower my patients to become self-reliant, I encouraged Dorothy to practice the Resist and Desire process on her own, which is a crucial part of the NPR protocol. This enabled her to realize that the emotional abuse she'd experienced in childhood seeded the unconscious expectation that she would be treated exactly the same way for the rest of her life.

As an adult, she unwittingly created or entered situations in which she would be emotionally abused, and her physical ailments were continuous. Once her underlying emotions were revealed, however, she felt that the next natural step was for her to release them and heal.

This chapter teaches you how to practice the Resist and Desire process on your own. The basic tenets of the NPR protocol, as well as its effectiveness as a therapy, are supported by extensive scientific evidence suggesting that your emotions, beliefs, and self-images can burden the immune system so that you become vulnerable to allergies, multiple chemical sensitivities, depression, and more. (For information on research that validates NPR's effectiveness, see appendix B.)

While the foundation of the NPR protocol stems from the Five Element Theory, it incorporates homeopathic remedies, which are used to detoxify the old sabotaging identities and belief systems that can cause illness. First, we locate the beliefs and the identities that have become stuck (through resisting them for years) in an organ or a gland. Then we perform the Resist and Desire process to neutralize the identity. Finally, we use a homeopathic remedy to detoxify the emotion, the belief, and the identity. You'll find homeopathic remedies for specific emotions in chapter 7.

NPR's effectiveness is buttressed by a large body of scientific evidence suggesting that it is entirely possible to *unburden* your mind and immune system from hobbling emotions, beliefs, and self-images. The area of science that embodies this evidence is called psychoneuroimmunology (PNI).

Psychoneuroimmunology

The fascinating and relatively new field of psychoneuroimmunology (PNI) grew out of groundbreaking work done by several scientists, including the Canadian stress researcher Hans Selye. PNI posits that there is a three-branched pathway by which mental attitudes and emotional responses can affect physical functioning and produce illness. Here is how PNI came to be.

In the 1960s, the psychiatrist George Solomon of Stanford University found that when he removed the hypothalamuses from rats, their immune functions crashed. Ten years later, Robert Ader at the University of Rochester discovered that the cells of the immune system, which were long thought to comprise an autonomous defense system, can in fact be coached to behave in specialized ways.

At the same time, Candace Pert, Ph.D., at Johns Hopkins University, was proving that similar receptors for the short-chain proteins called peptides live on cell walls in both the brain and the immune system.

While Dr. Solomon revealed that the hypothalamus critically controls immunity, Dr. Ader's work illustrated how the mind, most likely acting through the hypothalamus, can modulate immune system functions. Dr. Pert's work identified peptides as the communications managers between brain cells and immune system cells. Dr. Ader named this new science psychoneuroimmunology to highlight the mind, the brain, and the immune system connections that it described.

PNI connects the dots between stress and thoughts, feelings and physical functioning. It also maps links between the mind and the emotions it produces, and three of the body's most important regulatory systems, the autonomic nervous, endocrine, and immune systems. Extensive PNI research indicates that emotions, stressors, and how we interpret and deal with them can be a cause of such conditions as cancer, allergies, and depression.

The theory behind PNI puts you in the driver's seat on the road to emotional recovery. Only you can control what you think, and PNI research provides clear evidence of the mind/body connection and how we can use that connection to steer the body back to health. Many researchers, physicians, and psychiatrists lay the blame for recurring illness on patients by believing in the disease-prone personality. PNI research, however, suggests that this concept is erroneous and does not, in fact, exist. (So much for hypochondria!)

Instead, PNI holds that an *immuno-suppression/dysfunction-prone pattern* forms in the body and stays there. This pattern, to a large degree, determines how a person reacts to life events, which in turn affects the immune system's ability to resist disease.

I want to stress that people are never to blame for their illnesses. One of the most empowering findings of PNI, though, is that we need never be held hostage by our personality or our circumstances. In fact, we really can create our own realities. The path-finding psychiatrist Carl Jung repeatedly observed how we unconsciously create identities for ourselves, starting in childhood, by conducting ongoing internal monologues that prevent us from creating harmony in our lives or reaching our full potential. Many of my patients are so inspired by PNI evidence that we can improve immune function by changing our thoughts that they want to learn NPR immediately! That's what I call empowerment.

If you have experienced chronic emotional or physical problems, take heart. You really can shift your mind and body out of illness-creating modes that contribute to hormone imbalances and other problems.

As Deepak Chopra eloquently observes in *Ageless Body, Timeless Mind*, "The revolution we call mind-body medicine was based on this simple discovery: Wherever thought goes, a chemical goes with it. This insight has turned into a powerful tool that allows us to understand, for example, why recent widows are twice as likely to develop breast cancer, and why the chronically depressed are four times more likely to get sick. In both cases, distressed mental states get converted into the bio-chemicals that create disease."

The good news for you is that the same chemical connection to emotions described by Dr. Chopra conveys the health benefits of positive thoughts to the autonomic nervous, the endocrine, and the immune systems. Trust, joy, love, and laughter all reward the body by inducing the relaxation response and secreting chemicals that boost immunity and make you feel stronger and more youthful. Here are some things that you can start doing now to increase PNI support in your mind and body.

- Integrate relaxation techniques in your life, such as breathing connected breaths for five minutes.

- Create visualizations that are linked to self-healing. For example, learn as much as possible about the physical condition you have and then imagine those tumors, fibroids, or cysts shrinking like a deflating balloon. (You can do this with any health challenge.)

- Engage in simple meditations. Meditation stops the mind's awareness of its surroundings and refocuses the mind on a single thought. This exercise temporarily relieves the body of the barrage of chemical reactions generated by thought processes, thus providing a temporary reprieve from stress.

- Get rid of your limiting beliefs and self-images by experiencing the Resist and Desire neutralization process that is described later in this chapter.

- Develop the imaginative right brain to become more creative and idealistic. Read imagination-stimulating books to open the mind to new possibilities. Practice hobbies to encourage creative expression.

Understanding Your Emotional Perspective

Keeping the remarkable healing insights of PNI in mind, the next logical step in learning how to heal your emotions concerns mining the content of your emotions, beliefs, and self-images with honesty, compassion, and care, while also taking responsibility for them. The last step involves acting to change them from within.

For example, many aging people desire youth. If they look for it outside of themselves, they are abdicating responsibility for staying young, as well as misplacing their trust. Youth is a state of mind, and your state of mind determines your reality.

By now, you understand that your energy, emotions, and beliefs can either maintain health or create disease. What you believe is fueled by a conscious or unconscious self-image that could even be genetic in origin. Total wellness requires change, which in turn leads to evolutionary progress. If you resist change, the resistance itself can virtually cause illness because you become *stuck*. A chronic emotional pattern can lead to a burdened immune system and thus disease.

Have you ever examined the emotional perspective that colors your behavior toward yourself and others? I urge you to reflect on this for a few minutes and write down ten situations, people, issues, or events that you resist experiencing in your life. This means you'll write down the things you prefer not to interact with or examine closely. As my patients have found, doing this exercise lights the dark corners of your personality and provides new insights on how and why you manifest illness or unhappiness. Remember, the perspective that you live with is the perspective that creates your experiences.

Over the last twenty years, I've helped many people break out of the emotionally dark and negative spaces that they called home. Here is the formula that I recommend to my patients for emerging into the emotional light.

1. Consciously and willingly take responsibility for your experiences by examining and lightening your emotional perspectives and mental beliefs, using the tools detailed in this chapter.

2. Next, change the areas in your life that are crying out for it, such as diet, nutrition, emotional work, and physical exercise. Detoxification methods, especially for the liver and for heavy metals, are also essential steps to take.

3. Educate yourself about your body, including your individual hormones. Take notes. Treat your body like the best friend that it truly is.

4. Implement a nontoxic, natural way to correct emotional and hormonal issues through the detoxification of mind, emotions, and physical body.

One of the most valuable tools that you can use toward this worthy goal of overcoming negativity is the exquisite method of emotional healing contained within the Five Element Theory.

The Five Element Guide to Understanding Emotions and Health Problems

As I mentioned in chapter 2, the traditional Chinese Five Element Theory is relevant to your health because this nature-based system is a remarkably nuanced way to evaluate and improve your emotional, physical, and spiritual health. The Five Element Theory emerged during the Warring States period in China, between 476 and 221 B.C.

During this time, a school of philosophy developed that was labeled the Naturalist School. Students of this philosophy studied and interpreted interrelationships between people and their natural surroundings. They were forerunners of present-day naturopathic doctors and acupuncturists.

The Five Element Theory holds that by observing the flow of nature's energy from season to season, we can understand the checks and balances that are present in our own bodies at a given time. The theory maintains that what's true in the environment in which we live is also true within our bodies.

While the Western physician separates the various organs and functions of the body into different systems and categories, in Five Element Theory acupuncture, our state is viewed from a larger perspective, as one would view an ecosystem: no single part can be fully understood without an understanding of the whole. By hearing, seeing, smelling, and feeling, a well-trained Five Element acupuncturist can interpret which of the elements is your unique causative factor and on which level of the body-mind-spirit to focus.

Each of the Five Elements of water, wood, fire, earth, and metal correlates to a particular season, color, sound, odor, emotion, tissue type, time of day, climate, organ function, and other details that contribute to an understanding of the person who demonstrates an affinity with the given element.

As in all natural systems, each element feeds the next and is dependent upon it, just as in a mother–child relationship. For example, if an ailing mother cannot nourish her crying child, simply treating the symptom (satisfying the child's immediate needs) will never correct the causative factor (the emotional and mental concerns of the mother, the source). A Five Element acupuncturist seeks to locate the source, to balance and strengthen the energy where it is weak, and the symptoms in turn become resolved.

You're going to become your own detective and healer, using the Five Element Theory. You'll use it to locate the emotional causes of your health issues. Then you can find the homeopathic remedy in chapter 7 to help you let the emotion go.

As I alluded to earlier in this chapter, emotional traumas and mental causes of our symptoms can lodge in our bodies when we are very young children.

Resisted emotions not only reside in organs and glands (according to Traditional Chinese Medicine), but also get stuck in muscles, causing aches, pain, stress, and tension.

The Five Elements is an extremely accurate method of diagnosis, and you can use it in the privacy of your own home. A fascinating attribute of this theory will help you connect your health dots. Since more than one organ and emotion is related to an element, they can easily affect each other. Therefore, when you have a health problem with your lungs (grief), like bronchitis, pneumonia, or asthma, your colon (stuck) is at risk of dysfunction.

Alternatively, a health issue that starts in the colon can create a cough, bronchitis, and more. By reviewing the Five Element Chart and the description of each of the following elements, you'll be able to connect your symptoms to times of day and night and to the corresponding organs and emotions. In short, you'll have a big-picture sense of your health and the unique and precious ecosystem of your mind, body, and spirit.

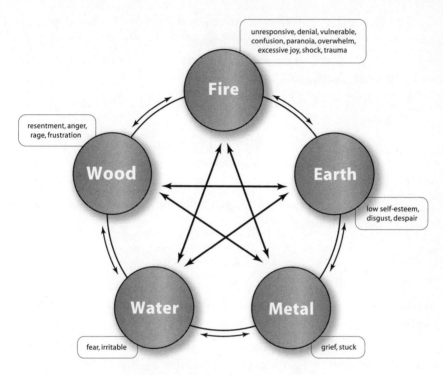

FIGURE 4: FIVE ELEMENT EMOTIONS CHART

The Fire Element

Organs	Emotions	Exact Time
heart	feeling overwhelmed, trauma, shock, and guilt	noon
small intestines	vulnerability	2:00 P.M.
sex circulation	denial and unresponsiveness	8:00 P.M.
thyroid and adrenal	anxiety, confusion, and paranoia	10:00 P.M.

Fire is the element of summer and is associated with the emotion of joy. Fire people love to reach out and be in relationship with everyone. They enjoy laughing, yet sometimes they carry sadness or a lack of joy deep within themselves.

The fire element has many corresponding organs, glands, and emotions. These are:

The heart: The emotions that affect the heart are shock, trauma, excessive joy, feeling overwhelmed, and guilt. (I discovered that guilt is related to the fire element by testing thousands of people with heart conditions.)

The small intestines: The emotion related to this organ is vulnerability.

The thyroid and adrenal glands: The emotions related to these two glands are confusion and/or paranoia.

The endocrine system (female and male): The emotion for both men and women that's related to the endocrine system is being in denial or being unresponsive.

The Earth Element

Organs	Emotions	Exact Time
stomach	disgust, despair, depression	8:00 A.M.
spleen and pancreas	low self-esteem, rejection	10:00 A.M.

Earth is the element of late summer and is associated with the emotion of sympathy. Earth people have the ability to nourish, as a mother can nourish a child. Thus, food and understanding are important. Sometimes an earth person can feel a sense of emptiness or neediness in his or her life.

The emotions and the organs related to this element are:

The spleen and the pancreas: The emotion for both of these is low *self-esteem/rejection.*

The stomach: The emotion for this is disgust and/or despair, which creates depression.

The Metal Element

Organs	Emotions	Exact Time
lungs	grief	4:00 A.M.
large intestines	stuck in a behavioral pattern	6:00 A.M.

There are two organs and two emotions in the metal element. The organs are the lungs and the colon.

Metal is the element of autumn and is associated with grief. Metal people search for what is pure and spiritual. They set the highest standards for themselves and others, and respect is crucial. Sometimes they live with too strong a sense of what could have been, rather than what actually is.

The lungs are associated with grief.

The colon is associated with being stuck in some behavioral pattern or belief system.

The Water Element

Organs	Emotions	Exact Time
kidneys	fear	6:00 P.M.
bladder	irritation	4:00 P.M.

Water is the element of winter and is associated with the emotion fear. Water people have persistence and determination and will often excel in situations that others find too scary. Sometimes they may hide a deep sense of being frozen or washed away by their own fear.

The kidneys are related to the emotion fear.

The bladder is related to the emotion irritation.

The Wood Element

Organs	Emotions	Exact Time
gallbladder	resentment	midnight
liver	anger, rage, frustration	2:00 A.M.

Wood is the element of spring and is associated with the emotion anger. Wood people excel or have trouble in planning, decisions, and action.

The future and their ability to see it can be their strength. When out of balance, they may procrastinate or lack hope.

The liver is related to the emotions anger, rage, and frustration.

The gallbladder is related to the emotion resentment.

Now that you know how to use the Five Elements to help you interpret your emotional and physical condition, you're ready to learn the specifics about your emotional state. Whenever we detoxify and heal, but especially when we try to balance our hormones, we must always remember to focus on the part of ourselves that we tend to resist the most: our emotions.

I know from more than twenty years of helping patients that excavating one's emotional life can be, at best, challenging and, at worst, downright traumatic. Yet profound self-acceptance and healing wisdom can come from our stating troublesome emotional issues openly and with compassion for ourselves. Toward that end, take the following Neuro-Emotional Assessment Test to help you identify the emotions that you need to release.

This simple test will reveal the percentage of time per week that you feel certain emotions and which ones are more dominant. When you've completed your test, think about how much time per week you spend clinging to resisted emotions and what a relief it will be when you let them go.

If you're like me, you're concerned with wise time management. My patients often report that this test is an invaluable step in freeing up a lot of time and energy. By answering the following questions, you'll become aware of where you are holding resisted emotions, stress, and potential illness in your body. Check off the emotions and the percentage of time per week that you experience them.

(For example, if you feel irritated half the day, seven days a week, write down 50 percent, and so on.) When you're done, compare your answers to the information that relates emotions to specific organs.

Neuro-Emotional Self-Assessment Test

Check here what percent of the time you feel this way.

☐ 1. Irritated _____%
☐ 2. Resentment _____%
☐ 3. Shock ☐ Trauma _____%
          ☐ Unrequited Love _____%
          ☐ Overwhelmed _____%
          ☐ Guilt _____%
☐ 4. Fear _____%
☐ 5. Stuck _____%
    ☐ Holding onto _____%
☐ 6. Anger _____%
    ☐ Frustration _____%
☐ 7. Grief _____%
☐ 8. Vulnerability _____%

- [ ] 9. Low Self-Esteem _____%
    - [ ] Rejection _____%
- [ ] 10. Disgust _____%
    - [ ] Despair _____%
- [ ] 11. Confusion _____%
    - [ ] Paranoia _____%
- [ ] 12. Male—Reproductive _____%
    - [ ] Unresponsive/Denial _____%
- [ ] 13. Female—Reproductive _____%
    - [ ] Unresponsive/Denial _____%

When you read chapter 7, you'll see homeopathic remedies listed for the emotions that you've indicated on the test. Consult the homeopathic chart in chapter 7 for remedies that may apply to your condition. Now that you've gained more useful information about your inner life, here's another healing model to help you manage your emotions even more skillfully.

Embracing Our Internal and External Dragons

According to the late Professor J. F. Worsley, who created Classical Five Element (Worsley) Acupuncture, we can be plagued by internal and external dragons, or blocks, that create significant disruptions in the connection between our body, mind, and spirit. Worsley theorized that internal dragons have more to do with internal causes of disease, whereas external ones relate to phenomena such as environmental toxins or chemical or mercury amalgam poisoning.

A patient who harbors internal and/or external dragons may experience a lack of control over aspects of his or her body, mind, or spirit. This usually manifests as difficulty in communicating directly to another person, such as avoiding another person's gaze when conversing. It can also be experienced as an inability to access emotions or resolve emotional woes.

It's important to realize that much emotional balancing may be necessary in order to create vitality and wellness. Wellness is created through your mind and your perceptions, and, at one time or another, everyone needs emotional balancing. So imagine how I feel when people who are obviously wrestling with emotional conflicts assure me that all of their emotional problems have been resolved! See if the following story reminds you of anyone in your life.

I once had a boyfriend who had complex emotional conflicts. He constantly battled internal dragons, and this made our relationship difficult, so I broke it off. Seventeen years later, we met up again. Although he still exhibited some of the troubled behavior that had compelled me to leave him, he claimed that he'd resolved all of his problems by going to a psychiatrist for two years. Surprised, I replied, "You fixed all of your emotional and mental problems in only two years by speaking with a shrink?"

His chest puffed up as he assured me that he had no more emotional issues or negative emotional reactions. "I learned that everything that comes up now in a relationship," he explained, "is just the other person's perception, which has absolutely nothing to do with me." Amazed at his inability to understand or take responsibility for his emotions, I smiled with compassion.

I'd like to share a secret with you. It's impossible for a person with childhood traumas to exorcise all of the emotional issues that arise in a relationship in just two years, regardless of what method the individual uses. There is one overriding reason for this: we're human, and we constantly face internal and external challenges. Unless we live in a closet, we have interactions with people, family, friends, the government, various institutions, and maybe even the law. So, the best we can do is monitor our emotions with compassion and defuse them healthily, using techniques that include homeopathy and the Resist and Desire process.

The Resist and Desire Process

I've taught this method over the last ten years to both health-care professionals and lay people. It's part of my NeuroPhysical Reprogramming (NPR) protocol.

The relatively brief and simple NPR process allows you to release deep-seated emotional patterns in a matter of minutes. It also helps you learn how to neutralize negative thought patterns and stuck emotions. Let's discuss how it's done, why it serves your best interest to do it, and where you can do it.

First of all, you can do it anywhere, and I mean anywhere, *except* driving. If you're an expressive, passionate person like me, you may sometimes have a problem holding your tongue or saying what you need to say diplomatically so that the other person won't be offended. If I'm in a business meeting and need to skillfully manage my tendency to express my honest feelings, I excuse myself and go to the bathroom. I get into a stall for four or five minutes and do the Resist and Desire process there.

So, you really can do it anywhere!

Now that you know this, you need to name what is upsetting you, which is why you want to do Resist and Desire in the first place. No matter what it is, go ahead and say it out loud. Just in case you have resisted an issue so much that you can't remember what it is, I've compiled a hit list to remind you. Reflect on the following topics with compassion and a sense of humor. You may find that you have problems related to more than one of them. Welcome to the human family.

Resisted Issues: Greatest Hits

Your hormones, PMS, periods, or fertility. A specific illness, a certain someone, a stressful event, a life situation you want to change. Then, of course, there are the age-old resisted issues of money, feelings surrounding one's religious conditioning, sex-related problems, and career frustration. Unresolved traumas from the past, anxiety about the present, and fear of the future are also common dilemmas. Many of my patients report problems relating to their jobs, their bosses, their health conditions, their families, money, their past, relationships, their husbands, their wives, their boyfriends, their mothers, and their fathers.

I suggest that you write down on a clean sheet of paper all of the previous topics. Then note what feeling each topic elicits in your mind/body. Now, choose one topic and close your eyes. What do you think of when you think about this topic? Are you thinking or feeling anything related to the topic that you'd prefer not to think about? Write it down and proceed to Step 1.

Step 1: Seriously consider what's causing you to feel upset. I suggest that you have all barrels open on this one. Choose an upsetting issue that's tough to unload. For example, if your boss at work is rude sometimes and it upsets you, recall and focus on one time this has happened. Or focus perhaps on an illness or an event that you can't get out of your head. You'll recognize the right one by how much of a charge or how intense you feel about it. In other words, how uptight, snarled-up, tearful, or burned you feel inside when you think about it.

Step 2: Now *experience* how this affects you, and really feel in your core what negative emotions it brings up. Often we push these feelings away (this is resisting a feeling) because they're so upsetting. Basically, we hope they'll never come back. But this time just go with it, really let yourself experience the emotion fully without suppressing it. As you do this, do what comes most naturally to you: *hate* feeling this emotion, while you relive the event or your experience of this person. Go on, stay focused, and *hate* them big time!

Step 3: You will now win the Oscar that you fully deserve because you're going to *feel, feel, feel* (this is not a typo!) that you *love* the emotion, event, or person. (Loving or desiring it will take the charge off it.) Really love it and desire it with all of your passion. This part of the exercise often indicates how much a person really wants to get well. Several patients over the last twenty years have protested, "There's no way I can love that!"

So, if they don't bolt like a thoroughbred out of the room, we're in good shape. If they do resist loving the issue, such as having cancer, which they definitely don't want to love, we go for the gold anyway. The object is to melt the resistance to having cancer and detoxify it from the body, which simultaneously bolsters the immune system.

Therefore, I kindly but persistently ask them to continue feeling the resistance to loving the issue or the person. Their reaction is key to why they are ill. So, if you tend to bolt like a thoroughbred, relax and realize just one thing. *It is only a feeling. It is not you.*

Step 4: Now I want you to alternate loving and hating the emotion, the event, or the person. Start with *hating it*, and then move to loving it. Emote backward and forward as quickly as you can. The trick is to love it and hate it with the *same intensity*. So, feel the hate and then love the emotion, the feeling, the event, or the person with equal intensity.

Step 5: Finally, after you've experienced hating and then loving the issue or the emotion a few times, *feel both the hate and the love at exactly the same time*. Yes, feel them simultaneously and place both emotions in the same place at the same time. When you accomplish this, the original issue or emotion will dissolve. You cannot hold on to two opposites simultaneously for more than a moment. At this time, you can choose to take a few drops of a homeopathic remedy to facilitate detoxification of the belief, the identity, and the issue from your body. (See the Resource Guide.)

Step 6: I call this step Relief. Playing soft acoustic classical music to balance all elements during this phase will help you to integrate the new identity and expand the feeling throughout your body. Many patients tell me they get high from doing this part of the exercise. After Step 5, you will feel neutral. Now, you have a neutral space to create magic with. Choose a new champion identity for yourself to fill the space with a wonderful feeling. Ask yourself these questions: What kind of person would I like to be? How would I like to feel?

A new identity is a new persona: a hormonally revitalized, healthy, wealthy, and wise person; a self-empowered woman; someone who experiences peace in his or her heart every day; a loved person; a creative artist; a peace keeper and a leader; someone who manages his or her stress like a sage; a winner.

Choose an identity and feel how it is to be that kind of a person, deeply, in every cell of your body. Expand the feeling as far as you can. Stay inside this feeling as long as you can. Breathing deeply and slowly, feel the new identity in your arms, your legs, your toes, your fingers, and all your organs until it feels comfortable and you own it. Congratulations!

Uncovering Beliefs and Identities

If it's impossible to bring up feelings or emotions, no matter how hard you try, you may feel frustrated. Please don't worry, as it happens to all of us at some time or another, even me. To get you going, however, let me clarify what I mean when I say identity, belief, and emotion. An identity is a persona, a personality, what or whom you identify yourself with. Examples include a daughter, a sister, a wife, a single mother, a girlfriend, a survivor, a lawyer, a doctor, a teacher, a sick person, a bad person, an old or aging person, a failure, a success, a good person, a poor person, and so on.

An identity can be good or bad. We don't want to touch the good identities, as we're concerned only with the identities that make you ill or unhappy. A belief is something you hold to be true about yourself, others, the government, certain professionals, and the world. An emotion is a feeling, plain and simple; a reaction or a response to anything, such as an event, a person, a deed, a place, an action, or even a type of food.

If you'd like to practice an easy way to reveal identities, beliefs, and emotions, follow these instructions. Move to a quiet location by yourself, if possible. Get a piece of paper and a pencil and go to Step 1.

Step 1: Write down the word *fear* at the top of the page and a topic that you'd like to work on. You may choose from the list of topics in this chapter or use any other topic.

Step 2: Ask yourself: What would I have to believe to make me feel *fear* about the topic? In other words, if you're using the topic "menopause," what would "a person" (take the attention off yourself) believe about her life in order to experience fear about menopause? Write down as many beliefs as you can. The words come much easier if you start writing the sentence like this: "I believe . . . " and then fill in the blank.

Step 3: Now, ask yourself: What type or kind of person would have this belief? You're looking for the identity, the anchor, and a component to all disease. You may use the previous list of identities to spur your intuition. Write down the answer without judging it or thinking about it.

Step 4: Do the entire Resist and Desire process (exactly as described in this chapter) on each negative or unwanted identity that you find.

After completing your rounds of the Resist and Desire process, you will have neutralized your negative identities and, most likely, the root causes of some illnesses. Moreover, you will have experienced the liberating feeling of ridding yourself of negative energies and self-sabotaging thoughts.

Step 6 Action Plan

1. *What to Do*. Change just 10 percent of your patterns in each of the following spiritual, emotional/mental, and physical realms, and you will be happier and healthier.

Spiritual

Step 1: Start meditation the easy way. Do the Bliss Exercise in this chapter.

Step 2: Meditation and prayer can exist simultaneously. It's essential to connect with the Great Spirit on a daily basis. Take walks in nature; perform acts of kindness and generosity. Find ways to give instead of take.

Step 3: Create new conscious behaviors and actions that are good for your health, the environment, the planet, and the peace process. Remember, we are like mirrors, so create peace inside before you can expect to see it manifest outside.

Step 4: Remember who you are and that you are a *soul*. Communicate to others from this authentic place.

Emotional/Mental

Step 1: Still the mind by revisiting the Bliss Exercise in this chapter.

Step 2: Release old, outdated belief systems and identities that keep you from experiencing spiritual growth.

Step 3: Change negative thinking into positive thinking. Do the Resist and Desire exercise in this chapter.

Step 4: Feel your feeling, and release your stress. Deep breathing is a way of cleansing the body, so sit comfortably and breathe through your nose and out your mouth in deep, long, connected breaths. Feel any stressful feelings that pop up and watch them melt away.

Physical

Step 1: Exercise daily. Take a walk; do Pilates, yoga, or martial arts; go up and down the stairs a dozen times; and go to the gym.

Step 2: Balance your neurotransmitters with sleep, exercise, amino acids, and healthful organic foods.

Step 3: Balance your hormones by first following the recommendations in this book.

Step 4: Take the correct nutrients for your body; heal your digestive system and gut.

Step 5: Embrace organic foods; eat more vegetables and whole grains; drink more water.

Step 6: Drink one revitalization juice daily.

Step 7: If you haven't done so already, *eliminate sugar*. (This one thing will make you feel 30 percent healthier within three weeks.)

2. *What Not to Do.*

Step 1: Make no changes in your life.

Step 2: Never feel your feelings.

If you follow these last two steps, you will feel poorly, while making doctors very rich and filling the pockets of insurance companies!

You are empowered by the knowledge that the body can create illness from holding onto emotions and stress, and you've learned a winning method for releasing negative emotions and healing your mind and body—the Resist and Desire process. Now you're ready for the final step in my program. In the next chapter, I'll show you how to activate your body's healing response by reeducating your hormone system with homeopathic remedies, a safe and effective natural healing method.

Step 7

Powerful Hormone Revitalization with Homeopathy

Katie was a vibrant woman in her early thirties. She came to me because her gynecologist (my client) was on vacation. She had been bleeding for the last two weeks, even though she had already had two D&Cs, one fairly recently. (D&C is an abbreviation of dilation and curettage. This minor surgical procedure is usually performed under local anesthesia. During D&C, the cervix is dilated and the endometrial lining of the uterus is scraped with a curet. In Katie's case, a D&C was performed to stop prolonged bleeding; however, D&C can also be done to obtain tissue samples, to remove small tumors, or to remove fragments of placenta after childbirth.)

Tired from invasive surgery and weeks of bleeding, Katie was wary of using drugs to heal her body. She felt that a natural, nontoxic approach would be better and wanted to know if I could recommend a homeopathic remedy for her condition. I gave her my hormone saliva test, and, after reviewing the results, I created her program, which included a homeopathic formula to revitalize her hormones and balance all of them, especially her testosterone, which had tested low.

The remedy reeducated her endocrine system to do what it is naturally designed for: making hormones in age-appropriate amounts. Within twenty-four hours, the bleeding stopped, and after she followed my program for six months, the problem resolved itself. Katie was greatly relieved to have avoided another D&C, and her menstrual cycle returned to normal. Her experience convinced her that homeopathy could be an effective solution for gynecological and other health issues. Katie also loved the fact that it had saved her from another surgery, while costing dramatically less than conventional medical treatment.

What Is Homeopathy?

Homeopathy is the second-most widely used medical system in the world, and I can say from experience that it's extremely effective. Ever since the late eighteenth century, the British royal family has used homeopathy. Her Majesty Queen Elizabeth II and His Royal Highness, Prince Charles, the Prince of Wales, use homeopathic medicine. Top athletes such as the English soccer star David Beckham; Hermann Maier, the Olympic gold medal skier; and Kate Schmidt, a two-time Olympic javelin medalist, also use it. The singer Tina Turner, a fabulously sexy woman in her sixties, whose hormones are obviously in peak condition; the virtuoso violinist Yehudi Menuhin; and Paul McCartney are other luminaries who stay strong and vibrant with homeopathy. Historical figures who preferred homeopathy over other forms of medicine included Mahatma Gandhi, the writer Mark Twain, the industrialist John D. Rockefeller, and the poet Henry Wadsworth Longfellow.

Homeopathy is completely safe and nontoxic. Even pregnant women, nursing mothers, and babies can use homeopathy without suffering side effects, although you should consult your doctor if you're nursing or pregnant. Homeopathic remedies can also be taken with other medication without producing negative side effects, but I wouldn't recommend that you use homeopathy with any form of conventional or natural HRT.

Unlike so many conventional medicines, homeopathic remedies are never addictive. Once symptoms are relieved and resolved, you can stop taking them. If no relief is felt, you are most likely taking the wrong remedy or are canceling it out by consuming caffeine, which often neutralizes homeopathic formulas. In my practice, actresses, actors, and celebrities have sought me out for homeopathic healing. (I practiced in a Los Angeles office for more than a decade.) All of these people chose homeopathy because the remedies are natural, effective, and nontoxic, and support the body without suppressing the immune system.

Homeopathy has many supporters in the U.S. medical establishment, including James S. Gordon, M.D., the director of the Center for Mind-Body Medicine in Washington, D.C., and the chairperson for the Clinton administration's White House Commission on Complementary and Alternative Medicine Policy. This commission developed legislative and administrative recommendations for public policy to maximize potential benefits, to consumers and the field of American health care, of complementary and alternative medicine (CAM) therapies, including homeopathy; nutritional, herbal, and mind-body therapies; acupuncture; chiropractic; massage; and other approaches.

In his book *Manifesto for a New Medicine* (notes section), Dr. Gordon ventures to explain why homeopathy may be so effective: "Maybe the remedies resonate with the body's electromagnetic field and somehow 'dissolve' the patterns of illness that manifest in that field. Maybe they leave a kind of electromagnetic memory trace in the water in which they've been diluted; perhaps their extreme dilution enables them to cross the usually impenetrable blood-brain barrier and enter the smallest structures within each cell."

As it happens, there are five homeopathic hospitals in the United Kingdom. I have listed them all in the Resource Guide, but two very famous ones are the Royal London Homeopathic Hospital and the Glasgow Homeopathic Hospital. Homeopathy is practiced the world over with great success, and this chapter is devoted to bringing you the most important aspect of homeopathy: the healing homeopathic remedies for hormonal balancing and women's health issues.

Origins of Homeopathy

The timeless healing system of homeopathy was created by the German physician Dr. Samuel Hahnemann (1755–1843) in the late eighteenth century. Since then, millions of practitioners and patients have verified that homeopathy is effective, safe, and nontoxic. I would also like to note that it's registered by the FDA, while over-the-counter hormone replacement creams and other hormone-related products are not.

Homeopathy is inspired by the ancient doctrine of similars: the belief that "like cures like." Hippocrates, the Greek father of Western medicine, wrote in the fourth century B.C., "Through the like, disease is produced, and through the application of the like, it is cured." In fifteenth-century Europe, the great healer and alchemist Paracelsus also practiced according to these principles.

Dr. Hahnemann developed the concept of "like cures like" into a coherent and holistic medical science. He taught that disease in a person relates to the whole person (body, mind, and spirit) and cannot be separated into parts or organs. The term *homeopathy* is derived from *homeo*, meaning "similar," and *pathos*, meaning "disease." Equal or similar illness relates to the natural homeopathic principle of using the *simillimum* to effect a cure. All homeopaths aim to stimulate healing by perceiving the similarity between the symptoms produced by the substance and the symptoms expressed (or suppressed) in the patient.

Dr. Hahnemann was a humanist who found orthodox medicine unnecessarily invasive, crude, and toxic. His conscience was troubled by medicine's many flaws, so Dr. Hahnemann gave up a successful medical practice to earn his living translating medical works into German.

While translating a book by the British physician William Cullen, Hahnemann read that cinchona bark successfully cures malaria because of its bitterness and astringency. This mystified Hahnemann, as he knew that cinchona was sweeter than other substances that had proved to be ineffective against malaria. His curiosity piqued, Hahnemann obtained cinchona bark and experimented on himself by eating it for many days. To his surprise, he developed the same symptoms of fever, alternating with freezing chills, apathy, and anger, that characterize malaria.

Hahnemann concluded that cinchona remedied malaria because of its constitutional "similarity" to malaria. In other words, cinchona could, in a healthy person, trigger similar physical and mental symptoms as the illness for which it was a treatment. Out of this insight grew homeopathy, the original evidence-based medicine, which considers the totality and the biochemical individuality of a person, the chief complaints, the chronological order of symptoms, and the symptom depth.

Like cures like is the first principle of homeopathic practice. For example, if you feel heartache and guilt about a relationship, you would want to take a homeopathic remedy that is known to trigger heartache and guilt. This is because a particular substance (whether it's an herb, a mineral, or a diluted poison of some kind), prepared homeopathically, will cure the same conditions it causes when you eat it. Why? Because it's the *energy* of the substance, not the substance itself, that acts on your body. Thus homeopathy can work for all diseases, such as hepatitis, mononucleosis, sexually transmitted diseases, cancer, or the common cold.

The second principle of homeopathic practice is that of "the minimal dose." This means that the remedy is taken in a hyper-diluted form, sometimes diluted to an extremely minimal amount. The third principle is the concept of "the single remedy." No matter how many symptoms are experienced, only one remedy is taken, and that remedy will target all of the patient's symptoms. This principle also relates to the concept that one remedy particularly characterizes each person: that individual's "constitutional remedy."

Homeopathy resembles other forms of medicine, such as conventional allergy treatment, wherein the allergic substance is given in a small dose, and vaccines, where a disarmed form of the virus is given to bolster the immune system against that particular virus.

According to historical records, during the Austrian cholera epidemic of 1831 and again in the American epidemic of 1849, patients who were treated with homeopathic remedies had far higher survival rates than those who were treated by conventional methods.

In the early part of the twentieth century, homeopathy was one of several branches of medicine that were popular in the United States. In a number of hospitals across the nation, one could receive purely homeopathic care or a combination of eclectic medical/naturopathic/ homeopathic care. In 1900, 10 percent of all American physicians called themselves homeopaths, according to Harris Coulter's history of homeopathy, *Divided Legacy*. These homeopaths trained in twenty-two homeopathic medical schools, staffed more than one hundred homeopathic hospitals, published their studies in medical journals, and prescribed remedies that were dispensed by more than a thousand homeopathic pharmacies around the country.

Across the ocean in Europe and in India, the practice of homeopathy continued to grow and to heal millions of people. The homeopathic tradition grew particularly strong in Germany, where I trained for some years.

Today, homeopathy is undergoing a renaissance in the United States, where several impeccably run schools train homeopaths. There is also copious research in the medical literature on the use of homeopathic remedies to address specific symptoms, as well as chronic and acute illnesses. For example, research demonstrates the efficacy of remedies such as Rhus Tox and Bryonia (or common hops) in reducing symptoms of rheumatoid arthritis, and Oscillococcinum (a dilution of duck's heart and liver) in treating the flu. All of these are widely available in health food stores and homeopathic pharmacies.

As you may have noticed, homeopathy uses the term *remedies*, rather than *drugs*, to distinguish them from allopathic (Western) chemical drugs and crude drugs of origin.

Let's talk about how you can get great results from integrating homeopathy into your endocrine revitalization program. Many of the best homeopathic practitioners are lay people. The advantage the lay person has over the medically trained person is simply that he or she does not have to overcome the emphasis on pharmaceutical drugs or the disease etiology that has been tattooed into the latter's consciousness.

What Homeopathic Remedies Are Made From

Homeopathic remedies were originally derived from the following substances:

- Botanicals: herbs, roots, and flowers
- Minerals and mineral substances
- Animal substances: venoms
- Electricity, X-rays, and magnetic fields
- Hormones, drugs, and poisons such as agent orange
- Healthy tissue or secretions of the body and organ preparations
- Bacteria, viruses, and pathology. Using these substances in my practice has saved peoples' lives. I cannot understate the importance of learning how to use them. If you have a grave illness with no known treatment, you can try homeopathy. Medical records show that diphtheria was cured in the 1800s by using homeopathic

remedies. There is a homeopathic remedy available for practically every disease.

- Secretions or flakes taken from a person's skin, urine, blood, saliva, and/or mucus are used to treat skin conditions such as psoriasis, acne, boils, ulcers, or infections.

All homeopathic remedies should be made at FDA-registered homeopathic pharmacies, according to the simple procedure of dilution and succussion (vigorous shaking). Succussion is also known as dynamization or potentization. It may sound like succussion is complicated, but it simply involves shaking some energy into the dilution, or remedy.

Homeopathic Remedy Preparation

Here are the steps that go into making a homeopathic remedy from scratch.

1. A substance is dissolved in an alcohol/water solution called a tincture.
2. Then one drop of the tincture is diluted into 9 to 99 drops of alcohol/water solution.
3. This solution is vigorously succussed (pounded and shaken). Succussion is performed on every homeopathic remedy; it imbues the water with kinetic energy, thereby increasing the remedy's potency.

    One drop of this dilution is then added to 9 to 99 drops of fresh alcohol/water.

    It is succussed again.

    This procedure can be repeated, with each dilution increasing the therapeutic effect and the potency.

"The potency" refers to the number of dilutions in any remedy that has been prepared by using succussion. Although homeopathic potencies go from very low to very high, most beginners start with the X and C scale. Conventionally, remedies are made on scales of 1:10 dilutions and 1:100 dilutions. The 1:10 dilution scale is designated X, and the 1:100 scale is called C potency. A 12X potency means that the original tincture is diluted 1:10, a total of 12 times serially, with vigorous shaking in-between. A 12C means that the original tincture is serially diluted 1:100 a total of 12 times, also with succussions between dilutions.

The number of succussions required for each dilution is not necessarily written in stone. In fact some homeopathic physicians violently dispute the correct numbers almost as much as traditional doctors dispute the validity of homeopathy's healing powers.

Homeopathic Strengths and Usage

You don't need to become a homeopath to heal yourself. You can simply use this book as your guide.

I want you to know what the potencies mean so that when you visit the health food store or your local pharmacy, you have a general understanding of them. Low potencies are 3X, 3C, 6X, 6C, 12X, 12C, 30X, and 30C. You may use these potencies for physical symptoms, from an ache or a pain all the way to hepatitis, rashes, and menopausal symptoms. Low potencies are recommended for the elderly, weak individuals, and children. Higher potencies are 60X, 60C, 200X, 200C, up to 1M and above. (A 1M potency has been serially diluted 1,000 times.) Although a 30C potency can be useful for physical and emotional issues, depending on the patient and the symptoms, the higher the potency, the more effective it is for mental, emotional, and spiritual conditions. Both children and adults can benefit from high potencies.

Homeopathic potencies are made according to specific recipes. So, for example, a low potency of 12X is a recipe for a formula that has been serially diluted 12 times, with vigorous shaking after each dilution. Most remedies come in the potencies mentioned previously, or they can be custom made for you.

Approaches to Homeopathy

Let's look at more vital particulars of homeopathic practice so that you can better understand how the whole system works, and how it may benefit your particular conditions.

Classical Homeopathy. Classical homeopathy uses one remedy at a time in a rather high potency. Considerable time is spent with each patient to find the simillimum, or the single remedy.

Complex homeopathy. This modern approach is especially popular in Germany, Switzerland, and Holland. It utilizes two or more homeopathic remedies, primarily in lower potencies. It's often used in a fashion that is similar to orthodox medicine. For example, a liver complex of remedies is prescribed for a liver problem. This approach is usually disapproved of by classical homeopaths, in part due to the apparent emphasis on symptomatic treatment and the success that it delivers. Diverse remedies exist for conditions that include PMS, all endocrine conditions, arthritis, bladder infections, fever, candida, hair loss, and so on.

Clinical homeopathy. Another new development in homeopathy is using two or more single remedies, instead of just one.

Ultramolecular therapy. Homeopathy is often referred to as ultramolecular therapy, to differentiate it from xenomolecular medicine, such as allopathic Western medicine or herbal therapy. Homeopathic ultramolecular remedies have therapeutic potentials. Because these remedies exhibit clinically demonstrable effects, they're used in homeopathic hospitals and doctors' offices around the world.

Through the process of potentization or succussion, it is assured that the pharmacological (healing) power of the original substance is imprinted in the remedy.

Orthomolecular therapy. Molecules involved in this form of therapy are normally present in the body, such as vitamins, minerals, or amino acids. In many orthomolecular prepations, xenomolecular ingredients are used, such as binders, fillers, colors, flavors, or other substances that can exert adverse effects.

Homotoxicology: The hippest form of homeopathy. Around fifty years ago in Germany, a branch of medicine known as homotoxicology began to evolve. Homotoxicology, which is now practiced globally, means the study of the effects of homotoxins, or toxic substances, on human beings. Homotoxins are created in the body or come from outside the body; homotoxicologists believe that accumulated toxicity is the basis of disease. Accordingly, they aim to identify and treat the underlying toxic causes of ill health, rather than merely to suppress symptoms. What's more, they see all symptoms of illness as a demonstration of the body's attempts to eliminate toxins, and disease as the body's attempt to heal itself.

Examples of homotoxins may remind you of the many toxins covered in chapter 3. Homotoxins include mercury amalgam dental fillings, dysbiosis (unhealthful microorganisms in the gut, often due to an unhealthful diet, HRT, or antibiotics), chronic yeast infections (candida), as well as diesel and petrol fume intolerance, exposure to unhealthful electromagnetic fields, pesticides, and undiagnosed bacterial (salmonella) or protozoan (giardia and amoeba) infections in the gut. Homotoxins can also be foods that are irritating to the body, such as coffee, dairy products, or white sugar.

In minor, short-term conditions, the body can eliminate homotoxins all by itself. In more radical conditions, treatment is needed. If a homeopathic treatment is used to eliminate homotoxins, then authentic healing results. The inventor of homotoxicology, the German homeopath Dr. Hans Heinrich Reckeweg, dubbed this phenomenon *regressive vicariation.*

If the treatment suppresses the homotoxins, such as when antibiotics are used, then the homotoxins tunnel deeper into the tissues and rise again after a dormant period as a more serious disease. This process is called progressive vicariation, and it triggers chronic degenerative disease and, ultimately, according to Reckeweg, leads to cancer. He theorized that when a single remedy lacks the power to heal, it's because the disease has bloomed in such a weakened immune system that the person's vital force is too fragile to activate a healing response.

Reckeweg ventured that this could explain why in chronic diseases, where even the constitutional remedy was easy to arrive at, the response seemed minimal or nonexistent. Continuing this reasoning, Reckeweg believed that until the vital force or immunity is revitalized and strengthened, single homeopathic remedies may be unable to promote authentic healing. Therefore, a combination of remedies designed to enact various healing functions appeared to Reckeweg to be a superior alternative to help the body eliminate toxins and rebuild its defenses.

Homotoxicologists (including yours truly) believe that many chronic diseases are due to toxins that have lodged in the intercellular matrix. In other words, we believe that cells can be loaded with toxins, and that disease progresses when the body cannot eliminate these toxins. Symptoms may be nonexistent until the disease has a strong foothold in the body. The various remedies listed in this chapter can help cure acute and chronic diseases.

Homotoxicology always aims to regulate an unbalanced body. It usually employs formulations that contain measurable amounts of homeopathically prepared active ingredients. Homotoxic treatment has been used successfully in many chronic diseases and inflammatory conditions such as rheumatoid arthritis. I have followed principles of homotoxicology in my practice for twenty-five years, ever since I studied homeopathy in Germany.

Homeopathic Concepts and Terms

The language in homeopathic books can sometimes be archaic and radically different from contemporary terms. Should you wish to apply homeopathy to your health on a regular basis, you'll benefit from using a dictionary of simple homeopathic terms. Explained here are some of the terms you'll encounter.

The homeopathic drug picture. . A homeopathic drug picture is the symptomatic description of a specific homeopathic remedy. This is collected by testing remedies on healthy people, including their mental symptoms, emotions, thoughts, cravings, dislikes, and special sensitivities to environmental stimuli (weather, warmth, cold, draft, etc.). A drug picture also includes reactions to emotions such as feeling upset when someone tries to console you. This pattern forms the drug picture for a particular remedy.

Simillimum. The single remedy given should be the simillimum. Simillimum means that the patient's complaints and symptoms exactly match the drug picture of the prescribed remedy.

Materia Medica. A classical compilation of all the drug pictures of tested remedies or provings is used to determine the simillimum and other remedies. *Materia Medica* lists the remedy by its Latin name, in alphabetical order, and then describes the remedy's derivation, the history of its use, how it's prepared, and where it's collected from. The listing also includes mental and physical symptoms that are produced. William Boericke's *Materia Medica* is most popular. Others include those by Clarke, Kent, and Boeninghausen.

Repertory. This is a compilation of symptoms from drug pictures described in the *Materia Medica*, arranged in a manner where each symptom is followed by all the remedies that exhibit that specific symptom. By examining a repertory, you can find the simillimum.

Homeopathic aggravation. This term refers to an initial deterioration in the patient's condition, as a reaction to the appropriate remedy. Although the symptoms appear to change for the worse, the patient's general state of health improves. A worsening of the symptoms for a short period of time is taken to be a good sign that the remedy is working.

Drainage remedies. Drainage remedies provide good results in detoxification and healing. As you know, a major key to chronic disease treatment is good detoxification. Drainage remedies are low-potency singular remedies, which detoxify and regulate deficient or blocked organs and the lymph system, thus improving the quality of toxic elimination. Elimination of toxic materials occurs through our skin, lymph system, perspiration, urination, and bowel evacuation. Good elimination is the first condition that's necessary for quick and complete healing. Drainage and hygiene of the body are essential to correct and maintain health.

A drainage remedy will help you avoid homeopathic aggravation. Homeopathic aggravation (worsening of symptoms) may occur for a brief time, but the good news is that the worsening can be reduced or completely eliminated by taking a drainage remedy along with your main remedy. So, if you're taking Sepia for hot flashes, you might use a drainage remedy to help detoxify the body's lymph system.

You'll find an excellent all-around drainage remedy called Phytolacca (poke root) in the homeopathic chart in this chapter.

Right- and left-sided remedies. Homeopathic remedies are often indicated for the right or the left side of the body. Remember our discussion of cell phones and how they tend to mainly affect one side of the body—namely, the side where you hold the phone? Or have you ever had an ache in one of your breasts or ovaries, or all of your symptoms lined up on one side of your body? Homeopathy is such a nuanced science that its provings indicate which side of the body a certain remedy works best on. Thus, certain remedies are indicated for the left side of the body or the right.

So if you have pain that's more intense on the right side than on the left, look for a right-sided remedy to take, and vice versa with the left side of the body.

Substances that can neutralize homeopathy. According to the FDA Homeopathic Pharmacopeia (the official U.S. government–approved pharmacopeia of homeopathic remedies), the following substances can render homeopathy ineffective: caffeine, fragrance (essential oils, cologne, perfume, scented body lotions, eau de parfum, etc. I believe that natural oatmeal soaps or glycerine are safe to use during treatment, but stay away from all other fragrances.), X-rays, and radiation.

Hint: When traveling with a homeopathic remedy, use a lead-lined film-safe bag to protect it from harmful radiation.

Potentized medicine. Potentization is a process of increasing the potency of a remedy by dilution and succussion, on a special machine or by hand, enabling Hahnemann to evade the problem of negative side effects caused by the remedy. Part of Hahnemann's genius was to refine a method that allowed him to use the Vital Force contained within the medicine without causing negative reactions that were the by-product of the application of a poisonous medicine.

This Vital Force contained within the remedy was the primary effect on the patient's Vital Force. The secondary effect was the reaction of the patient's Vital Force when activated. In essence, the patient's Vital Force exorcises the toxic memory of the similar compound in the remedy.

If the minimum dose of the simillimum is used in its potentized form, the Vital Force of the patient can off-load its disease burden without a healing crisis or aggravating side effects occurring.

Vital force. The homeopath aims to quell the negative influence or disease with the remedy and by accessing the patient's Vital Force, or life force. The homeopath also believes that every substance in nature possesses a unique Vital Force, including each homeopathic remedy. Although he developed homeopathy as a science based on objectively conducted provings, Hahnemann remained a Vitalist, like the European alchemical healers who preceded him.

Serial dilution and other homeopathic manufacturing procedures. Three essential procedures are involved in making homeopathic remedies: serial dilution, succussion, and trituration. Serial dilution means that each individual dilution is prepared from the dilution that preceded it. For example, a potency of 6X is prepared from a 5X potency, and so on.

Succussion and trituration are methods by which energy is delivered to the homeopathic remedies in order to imprint the pharmacological information of the original substances upon the molecules of the dilutant, which is usually a 20 percent alcohol/water solution.

In trituration, insoluble substances are prepared with lactose (milk sugar), which is used as the dilutant, and prolonged grinding with a mortar and a pestle or similar mechanical devices is employed. This is a method of diluting remedies to achieve specific desired potencies.

Avogadro's limit. An Italian mathematician named Avogadro published a paper in 1811 hypothesizing an explanation to a puzzling rule of proportional volumes that was observed in chemical reactions of gases and vapors. Avogadro's hypothesis later became known in chemistry as Avogadro's Law. It states that equal volumes of all gases and vapors at the same temperature and pressure contain the same number of molecules. This law's implications were a breakthrough for chemistry, as they pointed to the concept of a standard number of molecules and a standard amount of substance. As it relates to homeopathy, Avogadro's limit means that a serial dilution of a homeopathic remedy beyond certain potency has no *discernible* trace of the original substance used.

This means that it lacks any molecules of the original substance remaining in the solution and will therefore be chemically inactive. This is why some chemists feel that it cannot work. They believe that if no physical substance is present in the remedy, it can't be effective.

Avogadro's limit is commonly held to be at a potency of 24X or 12C. However, this depends on other preparation factors as well. Most experienced homeopaths feel that the magic number is 23X, meaning that after diluting a remedy to 23X potency, there is no substance left in the homeopathic remedy, which makes it a very powerful energetic remedy.

The FDA-registered homeopathic pharmacy that manufactures formulas for me shared the mathematical breakdown of the actual substance that was left in a low-potency remedy. A 12X potency of any remedy still has approximately 1 picogram *per cc* of substance or molecules remaining.

Homeopathy Dosage Directions

Select the remedy that most closely matches the symptoms. When you initially start to use homeopathy, a lower potency (6X, 6C, 12X, 12C, 30X, or 30C) should be used. In addition, instructions for use are usually printed on the label.

Many homeopathic physicians suggest that remedies be used as follows: take one dose and wait for a response. If improvement is seen, continue to wait and let the remedy work. If improvement lags significantly or has clearly stopped, another dose may be taken. The problem with this method is that it may not work because it's the wrong remedy. Therefore, I mostly use complex homeopathy (more than one remedy at a time), a broad-spectrum approach, which also yields amazing and easily verifiable results.

The frequency of the dosage varies with the condition and the individual. Sometimes a dose may be required several times an hour; other times, a dose may be indicated several times a day; and in some situations, one dose per day (or less) can be sufficient.

To help you select the correct remedy, I have placed symptoms and the corresponding remedies for certain conditions in the Homeopathic Healing Chart. However, if you don't feel the slightest response within a week, select a different remedy.

Different Forms of Homeopathic Remedies

One of the greatest advantages of homeopathy is that it comes in several user-friendly forms, including tablets, pellets, or globuli; liquid oral drops and sprays; vaginal or rectal suppositories; and injectable liquids. I invented a new form called a transdermal liposomal cream that can be applied topically to the skin to balance hormones.

Inherited Toxins

Do you remember the discussion of inherited toxins in chapter 3? You can use NeuroPhysical Reprogramming (NPR), kinesiology, or electrodermal screening to determine the presence of these toxins and treat them with the correct homeopathic remedy and potency.

You may have to administer all of the homeopathic potencies to cure every layer of the suppressed miasm. For example, a patient whose testing revealed salmonella could test for the following potencies, which are administered over two to three months: 3X, 6X, 30C, 100X, 200X, 1M, and possibly even 5M potency or higher.

Using Homeopathy in Your Life

I've healed my childhood issues and physical diseases with homeopathy, even radiation poisoning from Chernobyl and a uterine tumor (possibly a fibroid). That's why I suggest that you explore homeopathy by reading William Boericke's *Materia Medica*.

Imagine all the fun you can have! You can research all kinds of personality traits and illnesses related to your boss, your best friend, your husband, your boyfriend, or your parents, according to their pathologies and symptoms. Just think of all the people you know who could use a personality shift! While you're at it, you can read specific remedies that are applicable to your own symptoms and shape shift your personality into a healthier format.

The wonder about homeopathy is that every disease has an emotional connection, and you can actually look it up in the *Materia Medica*. There may be several, and they're closely related to the Chinese Five Element Emotions Chart on page 175.

Lymph System Cleansing

We discussed lymph detoxification in chapter 3, and I want to remind you that when you use a homeopathic remedy to heal your hormones, mind, emotions, or any other condition, you also need to stimulate or move the lymph to get the toxins from the disease or the condition you're treating out of your body. Various methods, such as dry skin brushing and saunas, can help to clear it, but when you add drainage remedies to this regimen, you'll get even better detoxification results: healing will be 30 to 50 percent quicker.

Homeopathy and Designer Diseases

Thousands of women suffer from the so-called designer diseases Epstein-Barr virus (EBV), fibromyalgia, and/or chronic fatigue. They're called designer diseases because they have unfortunately become so widespread in the last twenty years that they are certifiably trendy. For this reason, I want to share my protocol for healing them.

How to Heal EBV, Fibromyalgia, and Chronic Fatigue

I'm sure that by now you know you must first address your adrenal cortisol imbalances. These imbalances can be created by stressors such as environmental toxins, liver toxicity, toxicity of any organ and gland, neurotransmitter imbalances, dental issues, and heavy metal toxicity. Emotional and hormonal issues are also contributing factors. (Parasites, microbes, viruses, and bacteria are not a cause but a result of a burdened immune system.)

1. You'll need to purchase a homeopathic remedy for EBV, fibromyalgia, or chronic fatigue, depending on your diagnosis and symptoms, in at least one potency, maybe two. The potency may depend on how long you've had the symptoms. I'd suggest starting with a 30C potency and then perhaps a higher one. These remedies are the exact frequency of the actual disease, so they work very well, as long as you know which illness you have and the diagnosis is correct.

2. Use an herbal antibiotic like organic oregano oil and black olive leaf, along with other nutritional healing methods, such as chapter 3's detoxification diet and supplements.

3. Hormone balancing is essential. Find out what your hormone levels are. Get the following tests performed: six adrenal cortisol tests, according to the Five Elements of Chinese Medicine Body Clock, along with progesterone, estradiol, DHEA, testosterone, thyroid-stimulating hormone, and melatonin. Then focus on balancing your hormones, using homeopathic remedies and the recommendations in this book.

4. Neurotransmitter balancing can be achieved by your undergoing a neurotransmitter urine or blood test and then using very small amounts of amino acids or homeopathic neurotransmitter remedies.

5. Check out your dental health. You may need to heal a tooth, perhaps one that has an abscess related to your symptoms.

6. Heal your autonomic nervous system by seeing a chiropractic physician. Cranial/sacral work is also excellent; the Upledger method is very helpful.

7. Follow a detoxification diet. Eliminate anything that is highly acid-producing, including dairy and meat.

If you think that homeopathy may never remedy your hormone imbalances or other conditions, have I got a case history for you!

I saved this one until now, because it highlights how healing homeopathy can be for women whose bodies have been profoundly stressed and weakened by conventional and bio-identical HRT—and hysterectomy.

Rachel was referred to me by a health provider. She exhibited adrenal exhaustion and had headaches and various menopausal symptoms. In addition to her eating disorder symptoms, which began to manifest one year after her hysterectomy, she had aches and pains and felt tired all the time. In an attempt to heal herself, Rachel had been taking synthetic and bio-identical HRT for quite a while, and when that produced side effects, she substituted natural phytoestrogens, as well as human growth hormone.

She said she felt as if her personality had changed, and that she see-sawed between happy-go-lucky and irritable and nagging. I used a combination of homeopathic remedies because her symptoms indicated that her body was confused and suppressed from using HRT. I put her on a nutritional program, along with complex homeopathic remedies, according to a comprehensive health profile. I did not give her a saliva test because she had already spent so much money on all of the latest antiaging cures.

I used NPR and discovered that she had severe toxicity in her liver; other organs were sluggish as well. I used homeopathic remedies to balance her hormones: Sepia, Sulphur, and Pulsatilla, as well as Oophorinum (homeopathic ovarian extract) and Lilium Tigrinum (tiger lily). I used each remedy in more than one potency and gave them to her to take home and use. For the eating disorder (anorexia), she took Nux Vomica (poison nut), which is an awesomely effective stomach remedy, in a 30C and 1M potency, along with Hydrastis (goldenseal) in a 6X and 30C potency.

Rachel followed the program and took the remedies for about two months, but within a week, she called me and told me she felt a noticeable improvement. She said that she felt more alive and could feel her energy rising inside. Rachel also did a gallbladder/liver/kidney cleanse, along with the detox program in chapter 3. She drank her revitalization juice regularly, instead of taking vitamins, as she had an aversion to pills.

I saw Rachel again one month later and she was eating two meals per day. Her hot flashes had subsided completely, and it wasn't long until she reported feeling totally back on her feet. After about four months, she told me, "I believe in homeopathy completely, because I feel whole again."

How Dental Problems May Cause Bodily Symptoms

The following chart was created from more than fifty years of research in Germany and other countries. This chart is essential for locating a tooth that has an ache or a pain in it. Use it to connect your health dots. Use it to see the organ/gland that is energetically related to the tooth, the crown, or the filling that's causing you pain. This

The Energetic Relations of Teeth (or Odontons) with Respect to Organs and Tissue Systems

Zones	I	IV	III	II	I	I	II	III	IV	V
Paranasal Sinuses		Maxillary Sinus	Ethmoid Cells	Sphenoidal Sinus	Sphenoidal Sinus / Frontal Sinus	Sphenoidal Sinus	Sphenoidal Sinus	Ethmoid Cells	Maxillary Sinus	
Endocrine Glands	Anterior Pituitary Lobe	Para-thy-roid / Thy-roid	Thy-mus / Post. Pitui-tary	Inter med.	Pineal Gland	Pineal Gland	Post. Pituitary	Inter med. / Thy-mus	Thy-roid / Para-thy-roid	Ante Pitui Lob
Sense Organs	Cavernous Sin	Tongue	Nose	Eye	Nose	Nose	Eye	Nose	Tongue	Caver Si
Tonsils	Lingual	Laryngeal	Tubal	Pal	Pharyngeal	Pharyngeal	Pal	Tubal	Laryngeal	Ling
Yang	Heart	Pancreas	Lung	Liver	Kidney	Kidney	Liver	Lung	Spleen	Hea
Vertebrae	C2 C1 / TM1 C7 / Th7 Th6 Th5 / S2 S1	C2 C1 / Th12 / Th11 / L1	C2 C1 / C7 C6 C5 / Th4 Th3 Th2 / L5 L4	C2 C1 / Th8 / Th9 / Th10	C2 C1 / L3 L2 / Co S5 S4 S3	C1 C2 / L2 L3 / S3 S4 S5 Co	C1 C2 / Th8 / Th9 / Th10	C1 C2 / C5 C6 C7 / Th3 Th4 / L4 L5	C1 C2 / Th11 / Th12 / L1	C1 / C7 / Th5 Th / S1
Organs Yin	Duodenum Terminal Ileum	Stomach Esophagus	Large Intestine	Gallbladder Biliary Ducts	Urinary Bladder Genito-Urinary Area Rectum Anal Canal	Urinary Bladder Genito-Urinary Area Rectum Anal Canal	Biliary Ducts	Large Intestine	Stomach Esophagus	Duodenum Jejunum
Jaw Sections	HE SI CS	SI PA	LI LU	LIV GB	BL KI KI BL	BL KI KI BL	LIV GB	LU LI	SP ST	HE CS
(teeth) right	1	2 3	4 5	6	7 8	9 10	11	12 13	14 15	16
(teeth) right	32	31 30	29 28	27	26 25	24 23	22	21 20	19 18	17
Jaw Sections	HE SI CS	LI LU	ST PA	LIV GB	BL KI KI BL	BL KI KI BL	LIV GB	SP ST	LU LI	HE CS
Yin Organs	Terminal Ileum	Large Intestine	Stomach Esophagus	Gallbladder Biliary Ducts	Rectum Anal Canal Urinary Bladder Genito-Urinary Area	Rectum Anal Canal Urinary Bladder Genito-Urinary Area	Biliary Ducts	Stomach Esophagus	Large Intestine	Jejunum
Vertebrae	C2 C1 / Th1 C7 / Th7 Th6 Th5 / S2 S1	C2 C1 / C7 C6 C5 / Th4 Th3 / L5 L4	C2 C1 / Th12 Th11 / L1	C2 C1 / Th8 / Th9 / Th10	C2 C1 / L3 L2 / S5 S4 S3 / Co	C1 C2 / L2 L3 / S3 S4 S5 / Co	C1 C2 / Th8 / Th9 / Th10	C1 C2 / Th11 Th12 / L1	C1 C2 / C5 C6 C7 / Th3 Th4 / L4 L5	C1 / C7 / Th5 Th / S1
Yang	Heart	Lung	Pancreas	Liver	Kidney	Kidney	Liver	Spleen	Lung	Hea
Tonsils	Lingual	Tubal	Laryngeal	Pal	Pharyngeal	Pharyngeal	Pal	Laryngeal	Tubal	Ling
Sense Organs	Ear Tongue	Nose	Tongue	Eye	Nose	Nose	Eye	Tongue	Nose	Ea Ton
Endocrine Glands			Gonad		Adrenal Gland	Adrenal Gland	Gonad			
Paranasal Sinuses		Ethmoid Cells	Maxillary Sinus	Frontal Sinus	Frontal Sinus / Sphenoidal Sinus	Sphenoidal Sinus		Maxillary Sinus	Ethmoid Cells	

206

chart clearly shows energetic relationships between teeth and meridians, organs, glands, and vertebrae. Moreover, if you have a dental problem like an abscess, you can easily see the relationship of that particular tooth to specific parts of your body. The middle of the table shows the upper row of teeth and, below that, the lower row of teeth. Follow each tooth up or down in the table to see its relationship to organs, glands, vertebrae, and meridians.

Homeopathic Healing Chart Instructions

On the next page is a chart that's designed to help you recognize your symptoms, so that you can select the right homeopathic remedies, potencies, and dosages. Please read it thoroughly.

There are thousands of homeopathic remedies. For this book, I've compiled the main remedies that are used for women's health issues. Please note that the dosages are much the same for each remedy. Since I can't be with you to test you on dosages, it's safe to take five globuli or pellets once or twice per day (more or less), depending on the severity of your symptoms. You can take more than one remedy at a time, and if you experience results, you may not have to take it for more than a couple of months.

Locate your symptoms on the left side of the chart, then go across the page to find the remedy and the suggested potency that corresponds with them. If you choose a homeopathic remedy in a liquid oral form, you would use 3 to 5 drops twice per day or more. You can make a homeopathic douche from any liquid homeopathic remedy; just put 3 to 5 drops in no less than 8 ounces of water.

For vaginal dryness, I suggest that you douche with a liquid combination homeopathic formula, which includes homeopathic remedies according to your symptoms, two to three times per week, until the vaginal dryness is completely relieved. If you have many symptoms and need more than one remedy to address them, you can take two different remedies per week, alternating remedies on different days of the week.

Homeopathic Healing Chart

Symptoms	Remedy	Potency
Vagina very sensitive Warts on vulva Severe pain in left ovary and left inguinal (groin) area menses scanty profuse perspiration before menses uterine polyps, fibroids overall tumor tendency history of vaginal warts HPV or gonorrhea cancer tendency polite but closed down; feel unlovable, try to live up to a perfect image feel worse in cold, damp weather and better upon physical exertion and warmth	Thuja (plant: white cedar)	30C
A powerful influence over pelvic organs, adapted to many reflex states dependent on some pathological condition of the uterus and ovaries menses early menses scanty menses dark menses clotted menses offensive menses flow only when active uterus inflammation or infection prolapsed uterus pain in ovaries and down thighs smarting in labia sexual instinct awakened	Lilium Tigrinum (flower: tiger lily)	6C to 30C
vagina burns offensive perspiration menses too late menses short, scanty, and difficult menses preceded by headache or have suddenly stopped nipples cracked, smart, and burn	Sulphur (the mineral)	6C to 30C
fibroids, enlarged uterus, painful ovarian tumors; hard swollen glands milky vaginal discharges; increased sex desire; dysmenorrhea; irregular, heavy menses; breast cysts; symptoms are worse at night, in the cold or the heat, but are better in the open air.	Calcium Iod (calcium iodide)	6x, 6C, 30C, and 1M

Homeopathic Healing Chart *(continued)*		
Symptoms	*Remedy*	*Potency*
uterine fibroids, polyps, prolapsed uterus; hard glandular swelling pressing down or cutting pains in ovary and uterus; spasms; negative effects of sexual abstinence; people who have an aversion to sex; cancerous tendency scanty menses that is worse at night, in the cold, and with motion; better under pressure or lying down gradually declining energy, mental function, and emotional life; paralysis breast tumors; enlarged hard breasts or shrunken, lax breasts; hard glands tumor at site of injury or irritation (along bra lines); stitching feeling in nipples progressive weakness, mental and physical; atrophy of glands effects of grief, overwork, alcohol, old age fear if alone; guilt feelings; worse in cold weather and at night; better with movement and pressure	Conium (poison hemlock)	6X to 1M
uterine enlargement, fibroids; heavy, large, pendulous abdomen bearing down sensation, prolapse; hot flashes and alternating chilling sensations dysmenorrhea; heat on top of the head depressed, nervous, and talkative	Fraxinus (white ash)	6C to 1M
menses too late and too profuse liver problems	Cheledonium A prominent liver remedy (also for gallbladder and bile problems)	6C to 30C
breast tumor at the site of or after injury to breast (blows, bruises, etc.) insomnia after 3 a.m. or wakes too early; weariness; soreness in uterus poor healing, keloids, varicose veins; pimples and acne; painful menses feels need to move; excitable but mentally exhausted; angry dreams worse from touch, cold bathing, storms, chilling; left side	Bellis (common daisy)	6X to 200C

Homeopathic Healing Chart *(continued)*		
Symptoms	*Remedy*	*Potency*
breast tumors hard knots or tumors in breasts, accompanied by stony hard glands hard swellings in muscles, tendons, varicose veins, lymph nodes, bone weak tissues, shown by cracks, fissures, loose ligaments, poor nails, scars does things quickly but not well coordinated or effective; fear of poverty symptoms worse in cold, wet weather; any change in weather can make symptoms worse; pregnancy; better after warm bathing	Calc Fluor (calcium fluoride)	6C, 30C, 200C, and/or 1M
breast tumors large-breasted women; tumors with sharp pains into side, tenderness retracted nipple, breast ulcers, or atrophy; problems in unmarried women	Chimaphila (pipsissews)	6C, 30C, to 1M
breast tumors nodular tumors; painful, full, heavy, tender breasts; stitches into shoulder homesickness; profuse menstruation; worse when urinating, during full moon, and at night	Clematis (clematis)	6C, 30C, to 1M
hot flashes at menopause, with weakness and perspiration, and possibly fainting; uterine problem feels cold even in warm room pulsating headache bearing down sensations in pelvic area; weakness yellow complexion tendency to abort pregnancy menses too late and scanty menses irregular menses early menses profuse sharp, clutching pains violent stitches upward in the vagina from uterus to umbilicus prolapse of uterus and vagina morning sickness vagina painful during sexual intercourse symptoms worse in damp or cold weather fibroma	Sepia	6C to 30C

Homeopathic Healing Chart *(continued)*		
Symptoms	*Remedy*	*Potency*
menopausal symptoms, including hair loss and exhaustion sad, indifferent to loved ones; low sex drive; sarcastic symptoms worse in cold, damp weather; feel better in warmth depression: use higher potency	Sepia (continued) (inky juice of cuttlefish)	6C to 30C
menopausal symptoms thyroid problems	Lachesis Muta (snake venom)	6X, 6C, and/or 30C
heavy periods with odor sore breasts vaginal itching before menses uterine polyps	Sanguinaria (blood root) A right-sided remedy	6X, 6C, and/or 30C
cancer of breast cancer of intestines cancer of pulmonary cancer of stomach cancer of bladder	Carcinosin Made from human breast cancer and other cancers. This is the main biological remedy in all stages of cancer treatment. It has preventative capability.	200C
uterine tumors fibroids; chronic enlarged, displaced, prolapsed, or inflamed uterus habitual miscarriage, sterility, bearing down sensations, dysmenorrhea chronic ovarian inflammation, cysts; menses either scanty or excessive depressed, self-critical. You feel worse in cold, wet weather. Rest makes you feel worse as well. You feel better in the evening.	Aurum Natrum Mur (gold salt)	6C, 30C, 1M, and higher
breast tumors, nodules, hardened breast during menses; sharp, shooting pains; cracks of nipples, retraction; mottled or puckered skin indigestion, liver or gallbladder problems; chronic constipation angry, insulting, cursing; thick yellow mucus from nose, chest, and vagina	Hydrastis (goldenseal)	6C, 30C, 1M

Symptoms	Remedy	Potency
breast tumors, nodules, thickened breast tissue; heavy, hard, tender breasts enlarged underarm glands; discharge of milk, blood, or pus loss of self-value, indifferent to been seen naked, uncaring; weepy cracked, sensitive, or inverted nipple; old scars, abscesses; overweight worse in the cold and damp, with motion, and before/during menses. You feel better after cold bathing.	Phytolacca (poke root)	6X, 6C to 30C
first stage of mastitis: sudden onset, intense pain, red, hot, swollen red streaks or rays from the center of the breast; sensation of heaviness, throbbing extremely tender; fever, chills, face flushed, pupils dilated; dullness inflammation during weaning; worse in the evening, at night, at the slightest touch or movement	Belladonna (nightshade)	6X, 6C
acute mastitis: hard, hot, pale, swollen, and painful breasts caused by a chill, pregnancy, breast feeding stitching pain, thirst, fever motion makes it worse better holding breast	Bryonia (white bryony) prevents mastitis after breast feeding	6X, 6C, 30C
ovarian cysts	Oophorinum (ovarian extract from healthy animal source) heals ovarian issues	6X, 6C, or 30C
any chronic disease, including cancer	Arsenicum Album (arsenic) used to detoxify a patient with chronic toxicity	6X, 6C
yeast infections of the vagina, with discharge resembling egg white; with a feeling that warm water is flowing out of the body from the vagina vaginitis nervousness sensitive to noise	Borax Vaginitis that appears midway between the menstrual periods responds well to Borax.	6X, 6C

Homeopathic Healing Chart *(continued)*

Symptoms	Remedy	Potency
burning and itching feelings in vagina before and after the menstrual period discharge from vaginitis is milky and acrid or thick and yellow headache before menses swelling, hot breasts chilly and stout perspires easily and feels cold craving for sweets easily tired by exertion known pituitary dysfunction known thyroid dysfunction	Calcarea Carbonica (carbonate of lime) The great Hahnemannian antipsoric is a constitutional remedy. Its chief action is on people with impaired nutrition related to glands, skin, and bones.	6X, 6C, 30C
vaginitis heavy yellow discharge itching and burning vulva symptoms worse in the morning warmth and rest make you feel better kidney problem liver problem anemia weakness burning in urethra mucus in urine	Kali Bichromicum (bichromate of potash)	6X, 30C
thyroid problems: hypo great weakness during menses irregular menstruation uterine hemorrhage ovaritis wedge-like pain from ovary to uterus shrinking of mammary glands weakness and loss of breath going up stairs a warm person who wants cool surroundings	Iodum (iodine)	6X to 30X
vaginitis with watery, thin, unpleasant-smelling, very irritating discharge vulva swells and itches symptoms may be worse in the morning symptoms may be worse when standing up infections more likely to appear before the menstrual period or during pregnancy	Kreosotum (beechwood kreosote) Kreosotum is a mixture of phenols obtained from the distillation of beechwood kreosote.	6C and/or 30C

213

Homeopathic Healing Chart *(continued)*		
Symptoms	*Remedy*	*Potency*
vaginitis with discharge resembling egg white vaginal itching vagina feels dry and irritated personality is reserved, yet feels very emotional inside craving for salt feels worse from being in the sun menses irregular, usually profuse bearing-down vaginal pains; worse in morning prolapsed uterus depression: for depression, use higher potency	Natrum Muriaticum (chloride of sodium) Salt	6X, 6C, 30C, or higher
yeast infections creamy white or yellowish discharge, which can be bland or irritating sore vagina labia may itch or burn emotionally moody possibly tearful wanting a lot of attention and affection vaginitis during pregnancy depression: for depression, use higher potencies	Pulsatilla (wind flower) This is a female remedy, especially for mild and gentle dispositions.	6X, 6C, 30C

dissolving of adhesions anywhere; scars from
  skin disease; keloids
hard scars; burning, painful, or itching scars;
  better walking in open air
breast scars after mastitis, surgery, radiation,
  ulceration; swollen glands
tumors, inflammation, ulcers, cancer, developing
  at the site of old scars
	Graphites
	(graphite)
		6X to 30C

breast inflammation, swelling, or nodules before
  menses
mastitis; wandering pains, changing sides,
  constantly sore nipples
milky discharge
low self-esteem
hysteria
fears or dreams of snakes
worse with touch and in the evening
better when supporting the breast
	Lac Caninum
	(canine milk)
		6C, 30C

Homeopathic Healing Chart (*continued*)

Symptoms	Remedy	Potency
not breast fed; a person who chronically needs support and nurturing; a person who wants to be nurtured and fed	Lac Humanum (human mother's milk)	30C, 200C, or higher
breast abscess, suppuration; helps expel pus; hard, swollen, tender thick or offensive discharges from nipple; ulceration; fistula; fever inflammation and cracking of nipples, burning pains; breast appears red-colored in center, rose-colored toward outside; worse in cold and damp weather	Silicea (quartz)	6C, 30C, 200C, and/or 1M
depression responsible, ambitious, workaholic; loss of money, respect, love, power life has lost value; meaningless; hopeless, despair; serious; fits of anger sense of failure; worthlessness; blames oneself; guilt; violent outbursts suicidal; cheered by thoughts of ending it; silent, brooding; forsaken worse at night and in cold weather; better at night, in warmth, and in open air	Aurum (gold)	30C, 1M, or higher
depression apathetic, indifferent, resignation; dull, can't collect words or thoughts lassitude; listless and weak; mild, passive; loss of appetite; chilly overwhelmed; causes include overwork, study, grief, broken heart, burnout, adolescent growth spurts speaks in short phrases; desires juices; night sweats; worse from sleep	Phosphoric Acid (phosphoric acid)	200C, 1M, or higher
idealistic, romantic, responsible; self-reproach, shame, silent grief loss, grief, broken heart, shock, fright, upsets alternating moods; weeping, laughter, rage; cramps, twitches, spasm irritable, worse from consolation; sensitive to touch, tobacco, coffee held back emotions, sighing, sobbing, lump in the throat, bites the lip depression	Ignatia (St. Ignatius bean)	60X to 200C

Homeopathic Healing Chart *(continued)*

Symptoms	*Remedy*	*Potency*

scar tissue
stony, hard, very white scars; keloids; cracked,
   dry, fissured, hard skin
prevention of adhesions after surgical operations;
   hard lymph glands
problems at the site of old scars; pain, infection,
   or ulcers; itching scars
hardening of tissue, joints with fibrous nodules,
   and adhesions
	Calc Fluor
	(calcium fluoride)
		6X, 6C

scarring and other aftereffects of burns, scalds,
   radiation; never well since
old wounds or scars that become sore, crack,
   break open, or ulcerate
adhesions and contractions of tendons,
   ligaments, joints; stiffness
warts or scarring removal of warts
keloid scars, itching scars
	Causticum
	(potassium hydrate)
		3X, 6X, 6C

thyroid: hypo or hyper
anemia, muscular weakness, sweating, headache,
   nervous tremor of face and limbs, tingling
   sensations, paralysis
heart rate increased, dilatation of pupils
rheumatoid arthritis
infantile weight loss and rickets
delayed healing of bones
severe craving for sweets
psoriasis
tachycardia
goiter
obesity
mammary tumor
uterine fibroid
	Thyroidinum
	(dried thyroid
	gland from sheep)
		6X, 30X, 30C

cerebral hemorrhage high blood pressure chronic nephritis vertigo difficult mental concentration confusion used in childbirth, both to aid in delivery and to check bleeding after delivery	Pituitary Gland (healthy animal source)	30X, 30C

Homeopathic Healing Chart *(continued)*

Symptoms	Remedy	Potency
repeated exposure to X-rays skin lesions, followed by cancer distressing pains changes in blood, lymphatic system, and bone marrow anemia psoriasis	X-ray (made in a vial containing alcohol exposed to X-ray) For any kind of X-ray exposure	12X and higher
anxiety, nervous tremors, restlessness, palpitation, headaches hates thunderstorms limbs feel heavy	Electricitas (milk sugar saturated with electrical current) For EMF exposure	12C and higher
depression brain fatigue poor vitality skin eruptions, acne with discharge spinal problems; anemia trembling, convulsive twitching, and fidgety feet are guiding symptoms in this remedy.	Zincum Metallicum (zinc)	6X, 30C, 60X
mimic mononucleosis with chills, fever, headache, and general aches endometriosis irregular menstruation mongolism	Toxoplasmosis (parasite found in the house cat)	30C to 1M
chronic gastroenteritis food poisoning gastrointestinal ulceration Crohn's disease gastric headaches ulcers Ileocecal valve syndrome	Salmonella (bacteria)	6C to 200C
flu-like symptoms general stiffness anorexia neurotic depressive person meningitis syndrome headache: eyes are heavy and sensitive to movements	Influenzinum (influenza virus)	6C to 30C

Homeopathic Healing Chart *(continued)*		
Symptoms	*Remedy*	*Potency*
chronic ovarian ailments uterine fibroids cysts ovarian growths acute carcinomas or cancers digestive problems	Medorrhinum (gonorrhea)	200C (may need 6C to 10M)
constant headache memory impairment asthma sciatica frequent abscesses hair loss swollen legs fearing the night fearing that one is going insane fearing imminent paralysis	Syphillinum (syphilis)	30C to 1M
propensity to catch colds arthritis acute rheumatism nervous weakness tonsillitis exhaustion epilepsy rapid emaciation	Tuberculinum (pulmonary tuberculosis)	12C to 1M

Healing Your Emotions

Here's a list of homeopathic remedies to help you with your emotional issues. I know that these specific remedies are effective because they're replicated in formulas that I've developed, tried, and tested for more than a decade (they are FDA-approved and registered).

Find the organ or the emotion that you would like to heal. The remedies listed after each organ will help your body release emotions in corresponding organs, glands, and meridians. These remedies assist in healing mental, as well as physical, symptoms. For best results, high-potency dosages may be used.

I suggest that you purchase a *Materia Medica* to read the complete drug picture for each remedy and compare it to your symptoms.

Please see the Resource Guide for contact information on purchasing books and singular and combination remedies.

Emotional Healing Chart

Bladder: Feeling irritated
 Apis Mellifica (the honey bee)
 Hepar Sulphuris Calcareum (Hahnemann's Calcium Sulphide)
 Baryta Carbonica (carbonate of baryta)
 Staphysagria (stavesacre)
 Thuja (Arborvitae)
 Pulsatilla (wind flower)
 Bryonia Alba (wild hops)

Gallbladder: Feeling Resentment
 Platinum Metallicum (the metal)
 Chionanthus (fringe tree)
 Nux Vomica (poison nut)
 Arsenicum Album (arsenic)

Heart: Overwhelmed, excessive joy, guilt, trauma, shock
 Aurum Metallicum (gold)
 Coffee Cruda (unroasted coffee)
 Crocus Sativus (saffron)

Kidney: Fear
 Argentum Nitricum (nitrate of silver)
 Berberis Vulgaris (barberry)

 Arnica Montana (leopard's bane)
 Nitricum Acidum (nitric acid)
 Solidago Virgaurea (goldenrod)

Large Intestine: Stuck
 Nitricum Acidum (nitric acid)
 Cuprum Metallicum (copper)
 Agaricus Muscarius (toadstool—bug agaric)
 Arnica Montana (leopard's bane)
 Baptisia (wild indigo)

Liver: Anger, frustration, rage
 Arsenicum Album (arsenic)
 Lycopodium Clavatum (club moss)
 Cholesterinum 30C (cholesterol)
 Belladonna (deadly nightshade)

Lung: Grief
 Causticum (Hahnemann's Tinctura Acris Sine Kali)
 Natrum Muriaticum (chloride of sodium)
 Ignatia Amara (St. Ignatius bean)

Small Intestine: Vulnerable

Pulsatilla (wild flower)

Sulphur (sublimated sulphur)

Graphites (black lead)

Hydrastis Canadensis (goldenseal)

Aconitum Napellus (monkshood)

Aurum Metallicum (metallic gold)

Spleen/Pancreas: Low self-esteem

Arsenicum Album (arsenious acid)—arsenic trioxide

Lycopodium Clavatum (club moss)

Sepia (inky juice of cuttlefish)

Chionanthus (fringe tree)

Stomach: Disgust and despair

Aurum Metallicum (metallic gold)

Hyoscyamus Niger (henbane)

Nux Vomica (poison nut)

Antimonium Crudum (black sulphide of antimony)

Sulphur (sublimated sulphur)

Thyroid—Adrenal: Confusion, Paranoia, Anxiety

Nux Moschata (nutmeg)

Belladonna (deadly nightshade)

Calcarea Carbonica (carbonate of lime)

Phosphorus (phosphorus)

Natrum Muriaticum (chloride of sodium)

Argentum Nitricum (nitrate of silver)

Iodum (iodine)

Thyroidinum (dried thyroid gland of the sheep)

Monitoring Your Newfound Health

Once you've completed this 7-Step Program, you'll want to safeguard your newfound health and vitality. I suggest that you monitor yourself by retaking the self-assessment tests in this book every six months. This may reveal to you the disappearance of symptoms you might have forgotten about since starting the program. Keep the results in a workbook. You will see your biological age continue to improve and your symptoms disappear.

Women are complex creatures, and many things can upset our systems. By monitoring yourself regularly, you'll also obtain early warning signs that you may need to redo one of the 7 Steps. For example, if you eat out often, it's very difficult to avoid pesticides and chemicals in your food. You may find repeating the detox part of the program quite beneficial.

Being healthy involves a permanent lifestyle change. If you have followed the 7 Steps, then you will have learned how to take responsibility for your health. By monitoring your health, you become the mistress of your own destiny.

In the next part, I share with you some of my favorite recipes. They're easy to prepare and can become part of your regular diet after you have completed the 7-Step Program.

Step 7 Action Plan

1. Remember, homeopathic medicine has *no* side effects and has been used effectively for two hundred years. It is FDA-approved and will reeducate the body to produce its own hormones, naturally.

2. Practice the stress-management techniques you learned in chapters 5 and 6 to still your mind. By using this book to educate yourself about your body and your hormones, you'll find the answers you need to help yourself.

3. Ignore the celebrity marketers who want to sell you HRT or any hormone such as DHEA, melatonin, progesterone, or phytoestrogen cream as an antiaging miracle.

4. Never take supplements or any substances long term without a health-care provider suggesting proper dosages.

5. Take notes on how your symptoms wax and wane so that you have a record of your health that you can refer to.

6. Take all of the self-assessment tests in this book every six months, and address the areas of concern using homeopathic remedies, diet, and good nutrition.

Part Three

Life-Giving, Healing, Hormone-Revitalizing, and Delicious Recipes

Eating delicious, healthful food is one of the highlights of my 7-Step Program. The dishes in this chapter are steamed, sautéed, and—my favorite—raw. Not only do raw foods require minimal preparation; because they're uncooked, they also contain all of their energizing enzymes intact. Raw foods provide the body with superior nutrition and energy, and you'll feel great after eating them. Many of the recipes here are from my own kitchen; they're simple and straightforward to follow. You should be able to find all the ingredients in health food stores or specialty markets.

Food Preparation

First, you need to stock up on appropriate cooking utensils. I use only CorningWare (glass), stainless steel, or Le Creuset (enamel-coated cast iron) cookware. These are the most healthful and least toxic choices available. Never use any kind of aluminum or nonstick coating, even if the manufacturer claims that the coating never leaches into the food.

Next, use nonporous stainless steel spoons, spatulas, serving utensils, and so on. For slicing and dicing, I recommend using heavy glass cutting boards. These are easy to clean and to keep free of bacteria. They also last forever, and chopping never leaves indentations or marks on them. Another benefit: their surface is nonporous.

Finally, always wash your vegetables to remove chemical and pesticide residue. A simple way to do this is to use a fruit and vegetable cleanser/detox solution, which you can find in most health food stores. Rinse thoroughly with purified water after cleansing and see the Resource Guide for more information. If you follow the directions, this method should also remove parasites.

Equipment and Gadgets

Most kitchens are packed with gadgets: processors, choppers, graters, and grinders, many of which we rarely use.

225

My busy schedule demands recipes that are simple to prepare and user-friendly gadgets that multifunction so that I need only to turn them on and off. My father was a culinary artist and a pastry chef who loved cooking, designing, building, and crafting spectacular creations like six-foot-high chocolate Easter eggs. He had scores of utensils in his kitchen. I prefer a more streamlined approach.

Bottom line: I've owned a Vita-Mix (multipurpose food processor and juicer) for over a decade and use this multitasking machine for creating soups (without cooking—it also warms the soup for you), juicing vegetables (every part of the vegetable or the fruit is used), and making nut butters. (Besides tasting delicious, nut butters contain lots of protein and beneficial fats.) You can also make fresh, wholesome fruit sorbet (no sugar needed) and natural puddings and can mix dough or grind coffee.

If you prefer, you can always get a juicer, but with these, most of the fiber is removed. On the other hand, the juice's consistency is thinner than the juice made with the Vita-Mix. It's a little thicker than water, and some people prefer the consistency of this juice.

Another excellent gadget is the Excalibur dehydrator. This essential gadget helps you prepare raw food dishes, whole-grain crackers, pizza crust, pie crust, and dried organic fruit. You'll find contact information regarding the Vita-Mix and the Excalibur dehydrator in the Resource Guide.

Stock Your Kitchen with Healthful Herbs and Savory Spices

Herbs and spices have various documented health-promoting effects. When you shop for herbs and spices, I recommend buying organic ones and especially avoiding those marked "pico-waved" or with any other euphemism for irradiated.

Here's a list of herbs and spices and how they can help to remedy physical conditions. Remember to use very sparing amounts of herbs and spices when you try them out. A method that works like a charm for testing spices is to taste your dish. While the food is in your mouth, smell the spice you're considering. I promise you, this gives you a keen sense of how well the spice will blend with the flavors in the dish. Bon appetit!

Basil: Fresh or dried. Helps the body assimilate amino aids, expels gas from the intestine, strengthens the stomach, relieves spasms, and excites the appetite. It's great in tomato dishes, salads, and sauces.

Cayenne and paprika: Stimulate digestion, and both are general strengthening herbs. Use them in small amounts to flavor sauces and bland foods. These are both irritants and can cause digestive problems if used in excess.

Celery seed (ground): Mild stimulant. Expels intestinal gas and increases discharge of fluids through urine (diuretic). Use it in soups, stocks, stir fries, and stews.

Cinnamon: Relieves intestinal gas, impedes some bacterial growth, and is a warming herb. Use it in punches, teas, cooked fruit, and baked goods.

Cloves: Soothes pain and relieves nausea, intestinal gas, and indigestion. It's used like cinnamon in teas, drinks, and baked goods.

Fennel seed: Relieves spasms or cramps, aids digestion, relieves intestinal gas, has diuretic effects, and loosens mucus in respiratory passages. Whole seeds are added to soups, sauces, and breads and other baked goods.

Garlic: Relieves intestinal gas, regulates the liver and the gallbladder, and is beneficial for the heart and the circulatory system.

Ginger root: Increases the effectiveness of other herbs, imparts a warming action, and offsets the usual effects of a cold; relieves gas and is a beneficial stimulant; promotes cleansing of the system through slightly increased perspiration. Peel, grate, and simmer it in spring water for 20 minutes, and you've got a delicious and healthful tea that will also help soothe a stomachache or a head cold. Peel, slice, or grate it and add it to stir fries, stews, salad dressing, sauces, Asian salads, and main courses.

Kelp: Abundant in trace minerals, kelp is a nutritional gold mine and a tasty salt substitute. Use it in soups and stews to kick up the flavor to a zesty pitch. It's also good to use when cooking dried beans, as it helps to soften the beans and makes them easier to digest. You can find dried kelp at the health food store.

Mustard seed: Both a stimulant and a diuretic. Due to its irritant property, it is a mild bowel stimulant and a gentle purgative. It's good for seasoning all kinds of meat and vegetarian dishes.

Nutmeg: Used in very small dosages, nutmeg can reduce flatulence, aid digestion, improve the appetite, and treat diarrhea, vomiting, and nausea. It can have negative effects in dosages that are not used for culinary purposes.

Oregano: Relieves gas, spasms, and cramps; exerts a calming, soothing effect; is an expectorant that strengthens and stimulates the stomach. It's commonly used in Italian, Mexican, and Spanish dishes and is a great seasoning for sauces, salad dressings, vegetables, and legumes.

Parsley: Expels intestinal gas, is a diuretic, aids digestion, and relieves spasms or cramps. Use it liberally in salads, stews, soups, and as a garnish.

Rosemary: This strong and clarifying herb relieves spasms and cramps, stimulates digestion, promotes liver function, and calms the nerves. *Caution:* It can be toxic in large quantities. Use it on fish and some vegetables like peas or spinach.

Sage, dried or fresh: Reduces congestion, expels intestinal gas. This strong herb tastes more like mint when fresh. It's delicious in bean or vegetable casseroles and stuffings.

Turmeric: Promotes the digestion of fatty foods and relieves intestinal gas; has some antimicrobial and anti-inflammatory activity. It's a staple of Indian cuisine; combine it with curry powder to make flavorful sauces, yogurt vegetable dips, and more.

Thyme: Aids in the digestion of fatty foods; relieves cramps; is a tonic for the stomach and the nerves; expels intestinal gas; is good for respiratory passages; and is antiseptic. Use it to flavor vegetable casseroles, salad dressings, and rice and bean dishes.

Creating a Hormone-Healthy Kitchen

I recommend that you check your kitchen for the following items and throw away anything in the following list. They contain various ingredients that are toxic and tax your endocrine system, thereby contributing to hormone imbalance.

You'll find substitutions for many of them in the Real Food Substitution Chart, which follows.

What to Throw Out

- Any product containing preservatives, including freshness preservatives, artificial flavoring, artificial coloring, BHA, and BHT
- Canned foods lined inside with metal. Organic canned food, lined with safe, nonporous material, can be found at your local health food store.
- Candies and commercial breads, because of the sugar, the emulsifiers, and the preservatives
- Chocolate, because 40 percent white sugar is added to produce semisweet chocolate. Chocolate also contains the stimulants theobromine and caffeine. In addition, the oxalic acid in chocolate interferes with calcium absorption. I understand how wonderful it can be to eat chocolate, so here's a tip on the most healthful kind. I occasionally eat organic chocolate sweetened with maltitol or xylitol instead of sugar. This never affects my body negatively, so I say that it's okay to enjoy some chocolate every now and then.
- Plastic containers for food storage, as they may leach plastic into your food, which, as you know, is bad news for your hormone balance.
- Your microwave oven, because microwaves destroy the nutrient value of food and emit electromagnetic waves that can negatively affect endocrine function.

Here's a list of real food substitutions that you can use to promote hormone health. I give this to all my patients to get them into the groove of the nutrition part of the 7-Step Program. Some of my patients photocopy this list and keep it on their fridge to remind them what to use and what to omit in the kitchen.

Real Food Substitutions

Please use organic foods at all times. Do not eat genetically engineered foods.

Omit	Use
aluminum or nonstick-surface cookware	stainless steel or CorningWare cookware
coffee, Chinese teas, other caffeinated teas	organic herb teas, cereal beverages
commercially hydrogenated peanut butter and nut butters, salted nuts	organic raw sesame tahini, walnut, pecan, peanut, and cashew butter, organic raw nuts and seeds
sulphured dried fruits	organic unsulphured dried fruits
red meat and poultry	tempeh, deep-sea fish, soaked raw nuts and seeds
snacks	organic dried fruit and nuts, raw seeds and nuts, fruit, raw vegetables, whole-grain baked goods
dairy products	rice milk, almond milk, sesame cream, hazelnut milk
all-purpose flour and cake flour	whole-grain flours such as organic rye, corn, oat, rice, or whole wheat pastry flour
commercially boxed cereals	organic granola or whole, flaked, or cracked grains, raw (soaked)
wheat cracker or bread crumbs	organic whole-grain bread crumbs, whole-grain flakes, wheat germ, or whole-grain crackers
white rice, wheat, or other refined grains	brown rice, buckwheat, millet, barley, corn, spelt, quinoa
sugars (sucrose, dextrose, glucose, barley malt, maple syrup, honey, brown sugar, raw sugar, corn syrup), NutraSweet, Equal, aspartame, sucralose, etc.	organic agave syrup and stevia
chocolate with sugar	organic chocolate with maltitol or xylitol, carob powder (3 tablespoons carob plus 2 tablespoons milk = 1 square chocolate)

processed cocoa	carob powder or organic cocoa
baking soda	low-sodium baking powder (aluminum free), 2 parts in place of 1 part soda
baking powder	low-sodium baking powder (aluminum free)
cornstarch	kuzu, arrowroot flour
salt	Celtic sea salt, kelp powder, vegetable seasonings, tamari soy sauce ($\frac{1}{4}$ teaspoon salt = 1 teaspoon tamari), miso ($\frac{1}{4}$ teaspoon salt = 1$\frac{1}{2}$ teaspoons miso)
supermarket brands of mayonnaise, high in saturated fats	organic eggless non-dairy mayonnaise or vegginase
distilled vinegar	unfiltered, organic unpasteurized apple cider vinegar, brown rice vinegar, balsamic vinegar
hydrogenated fats and shortenings, refined oils	unrefined oils are best, organic flax, hemp, coconut, and virgin olive oil are the best
white pasta or any wheat (spaghetti, macaroni, shells, noodles)	organic whole-grain pastas such as corn, oat, rice, sesame, Jerusalem artichoke, buckwheat, kamut, and quinoa
soda	fresh unfiltered vegetable and fruit juices, spring water, herb teas, raw coconut milk
herbs that are irradiated or contain preservatives	organic herbs and spices that are nonirradiated

Changing your diet from junk food to an organic, healthful diet may be a bit of a challenge at first. But I assure you, after one week of eating only healthful foods, you'll feel better and have more energy.

Cooking and eating are two of life's greatest pleasures. I invite you to have fun in the kitchen with these recipes. Eating these dishes will help you gain vitality and strength and, best of all, help revitalize your hormones.

Recipes

Raw Food Recipes

TACO SALAD

shredded lettuce
Mock Refried Beans (recipe follows)
Mock Sour Cream (recipe follows)
Guacamole (recipe follows)
3 tablespoons salsa
Bermuda onion, minced

Arrange a bed of shredded lettuce on a plate. Leaving room in the center for the Mock Refried Beans, place a scoop of guacamole in one corner, a scoop of salsa in another corner, and a scoop of minced Bermuda onion in another corner. Top with a dollop of Mock Sour Cream.

Yield: About 2 cups

MOCK REFRIED BEANS

6 Roma tomatoes
2 tablespoons ground cumin
1 tablespoon onion, minced
1 tablespoon garlic, minced·
2 cups sunflower seeds, soaked overnight
2 cups almonds, soaked overnight

Put the tomatoes into the food processor and thoroughly puree. Add the cumin, onion, and garlic and process. Add the sunflower seeds and almonds and process to the desired texture. For a creamier consistency, process longer.

Yield: About 2 cups

MOCK SOUR CREAM

1 cup Brazil nuts, soaked overnight
½ cup pure water
¼ cup lemon juice
½ plus ⅛ teaspoon Celtic salt

Combine all the ingredients in a food processor until light and creamy, about 3 or 4 minutes.

Yield: About 1¼ cups

GUACAMOLE

3 ripe avocados
1 onion, chopped very fine
½ teaspoon coriander
½ teaspoon Indo seasoning
1 tomato, chopped
¼ teaspoon garlic powder
½ can black olives, chopped
½ teaspoon cumin
¼ teaspoon cayenne pepper
2 tablespoons natural fresh salsa

Mash all the ingredients together and chill for 10 minutes. Leave an avocado pit in the middle of the bowl before serving to prevent the guacamole from turning brown.

Yield: 3 to 4 servings

MOCK CHOCOLATE CREAM PIE

Crust

2 cups sunflower seeds, soaked overnight
2 cups Brazil nuts, soaked overnight
11 dates, pitted

Combine the crust ingredients in a food processor and process until the nuts are broken down and thoroughly blended. Using your fingers, press the mixture into the bottom and sides of a 9-inch spring-form pan.

Filling

2 cups avocado, peeled and seeded
2 cups dates, pitted
1½ cups organic carob powder
1 teaspoon vanilla extract
prepared 8-inch pie crust
1 or 2 sliced strawberries, for garnish

Combine the avocado, dates, carob powder, and vanilla extract in a food processor until smooth and creamy. Spoon the mixture into the prepared pie crust and allow to set for 4 hours. Garnish with the strawberries.

Yield: 4 to 6 servings

SPROUTED GARBANZO HUMMUS

2½ cups sprouted garbanzos
1½ cups raw tahini
½ cup freshly squeezed lemon juice
½ cup purified water
½ cup parsley, chopped
2 tablespoons garlic, minced
½ tablespoon sea salt
1 teaspoon ground cumin
¾ cup organic extra virgin olive oil

Combine all the ingredients in a food processor until the mixture is the desired consistency. Longer processing will produce a smoother consistency.

Yield: 3 to 4 servings

HEARTY LENTIL SOUP

3 cups almond milk (recipe follows)
1 avocado, peeled and seeded
3 tablespoons garlic, minced
3 tablespoons onion, minced
½ cup bell pepper, diced
¾ cup tomato, chopped
3 tablespoons fresh dill
1 teaspoon sea salt
½ cup extra virgin olive oil
1 cup water
3 cups sprouted lentils

Blend all the ingredients except the lentils in a Vita-Mix or a blender. Stir in the lentils and serve.

Yield: 3 to 4 servings

ALMOND MILK

1½ cups raw almonds, soaked for several hours or overnight
3 cups water

Blend the ingredients together in a Vita-Mix. Strain off the pulp in a fine mesh strainer.

Yield: 3 cups

PIZZA

Crust
6 ounces carrot pulp
6 ounces buckwheat, soaked for 24 hours
6 ounces flaxseed, soaked for 24 hours

Sauce
2 tomatoes
2 beets
8 to 10 olives
2 ounces extra virgin olive oil

Toppings
tomatoes
red bell peppers
broccoli
mushrooms
olives
avocado

Blend the carrot pulp, buckwheat, and flaxseed in a Vita-Mix or a high-powered blender. Spread the mixture onto an Excalibur dehydrator Teflex sheet. Set the dehydrator at 105°F and dehydrate for 20 hours. Flip the crust over and dehydrate for another day. For sauce, blend the tomatoes, beets, olives, and olive oil in a blender. Spread over the pizza crust. Finely cut the topping ingredients and spread over the sauce. Serve and enjoy.

Yield: 1 or 2 servings

FRUIT PIE

Crust
4 ounces freshly squeezed apple juice
3 bananas
18 dates, pitted

Filling
frozen bananas
any favorite fruit
dates

Blend the crust ingredients together in a Vita-Mix or a high-powered blender until pureed. Pour into a round 8-inch plastic bowl, and freeze overnight. Add the frozen bananas and any of your favorite

Fruit Pie (continued)

fruits to your Champion juicer. Add some dates for sweetening to the juicer. Process through the juicer, mix well, and fill the crust.

Yield: 1 or 2 servings

FAUX TURKEY

(It tastes like dressing and turkey.)
   2 cloves garlic, chopped fine
   2 tablespoons fresh sage
   2 tablespoons fresh rosemary
   2 tablespoons fresh thyme
   2 cups walnuts, soaked for 12 hours and drained
   2 cups almonds, soaked for 12 hours and drained
   1 tablespoon organic unpasteurized white miso
   1 large onion, chopped very fine
   6 stalks celery, chopped fine
   1 cup parsley sprigs, for garnish
   1 cup cranberries, for garnish

Place the garlic in a food processor and process well. Add the sage, rosemary, and thyme, processing well. Add the walnuts, almonds, and miso, one at a time, and process well. Remove to a bowl and stir in the onion and celery. Place on a sheet of Teflex and form into an oval loaf shape. Place in a dehydrator for 6 hours. Remove and turn the loaf over, removing the Teflex sheet from the bottom. Dehydrate for 4 to 6 hours more. Garnish with parsley and cranberries.

Yield: 8 servings

PUMPKIN PIE

   ½ cup pumpkin seeds
   1 cup raw macadamia nuts
   2 avocados, peeled and seeded
   ½ cup raw agave syrup
   4 dates, soaked for 3 hours in 1 cup filtered water
   2 teaspoons vanilla
   1 teaspoon ground cinnamon
   ¼ teaspoon ground nutmeg
   ½ teaspoon ground ginger
   1 teaspoon sea salt
   water

4 cups raw pumpkin, peeled
1 teaspoon ground psyllium husks
1 cup organic raisins
1 Agave Syrup Nut and Date Pie Crust (recipe follows)

In advance of making the pie, prepare the pumpkin seeds and macadamia nuts. Wash the pumpkin seeds. Soak for 8 hours and drain. Dehydrate for 6 to 8 hours at 95°F. Soak the macadamia nuts for 8 hours and drain.

To make the pie, blend the avocado, agave syrup, dates with the soak water, vanilla, cinnamon, nutmeg, ginger, salt, and macadamias until smooth. Add the pumpkin and blend until very smooth. Add the psyllium and blend well. Let this mixture sit for 10 minutes and blend well again. Fold in the raisins. Pour into the pie crust and top with the pumpkin seeds.

Yield: 8 slices

AGAVE SYRUP NUT AND DATE PIE CRUST

1 cup almonds (dry)
1 cup pecans (dry)
1 cup walnuts (dry)
½ teaspoon sea salt
1 teaspoon vanilla powder (see next recipe)
1 cup medjool dates, pitted
¼ cup raw agave syrup

Prepare the nuts in advance of making the crust. Soak the almonds, pecans, and walnuts separately for 12 hours. Drain and dehydrate for 12 hours.

To make the crust, place the almonds in a food processor with an "S" blade and process until the mixture resembles flour. Add the salt and vanilla to the almonds and process well. Add the pecans, walnuts, and dates to the processor. Add agave syrup to the nut and date mixture and process just until mixed well. Press the mixture by hand into an 8- to 10-inch glass pie pan. *Note: The crust may be made ahead of time and refrigerated or frozen.*

Yield: 1 pie crust

Vanilla Powder

5 vanilla beans
½ cup soft spring wheat berries or hulled buckwheat

Place the vanilla beans and wheat berries in a Vita-Mix or a seed/coffee grinder and grind to a powder. Place in an airtight container and store in the refrigerator.

Plum Pudding

½ cup macadamia nuts
4 dried apricots
3 plums
¼ teaspoon sea salt
½ teaspoon vanilla extract
½ teaspoon lemon juice

Blend all ingredients until smooth and creamy, then serve.

Yield: 3 or 4 servings

Vegetable Kurma

Marinade

2 cups water
3 medium cloves garlic
½ cup extra virgin olive oil
1 teaspoon sea salt
2 to 3 tablespoons yellow curry powder
vegetable (your choice)
1 cup raw almonds, soaked
¼ cup cilantro
¼ cup parsley

Combine the water, garlic, olive oil, sea salt, and curry powder in a blender to create a marinade. Pour the marinade into a bowl. Soak any vegetables of your choice in the marinade for 24 hours. Strain the vegetables, reserving the marinade. Pour the marinade back into the blender and add the almonds. Blend thoroughly. Add the cilantro and parsley and blend at medium speed for about 20 seconds. Serve over the marinated vegetables and sprouted wild rice or sprouted quinoa. If desired, adjust the seasonings with additional curry or add cayenne pepper.

Yield: 4 servings

BELL PEPPER OR SUMMER SQUASH SOUP

1 medium yellow bell pepper or summer squash
½ medium cucumber
¼ medium red onion
1 tablespoon extra virgin olive oil
1 teaspoon sea salt
⅓ cup water

Combine all of the ingredients in a blender until pureed. Serve. *Option: Combine yellow bell pepper and summer squash in the soup.*

Yield: 1½ cups

REVITALIZING JUICE

This particular combination of vegetable juices will detoxify the entire body, including the liver. Make sure all vegetables are organic if possible; otherwise soak for ten minutes in water with one teaspoon of food-grade hydrogen peroxide or use vegetable detox solution from the health food store. Rinse thoroughly afterward with purified water. Use more dandelion (6 leaves) if you have a chronic liver condition or would just like to detoxify quicker.

3 stalks celery
½ cucumber
5 basil leaves
3 tomatoes
1 clove garlic
1 carrot
4 kale leaves
3 dandelion leaves (if not available, use collard greens)
½ red pepper

Combine all the ingredients in a juicer and liquify.

Yield: 1 16-ounce drink

Sautéed and Cooked Food Recipes

SALMON ROLL

This recipe is rich in essential omega-3 fatty acids, which are the building blocks of your hormones. It's important to use wild salmon, if possible, since farm-raised salmon is often fed soy and administered antibiotics and hormones, making it low in omega-3 fatty acids and high in omega-6 fatty acids. If you suffer from PMS or any other

Salmon Roll (continued)

inflammatory problem, you want to avoid too many omega-6 fatty acids because they fuel the fire of inflammation.

2 organic romaine lettuce leaves
2 teaspoons sugarless high omega-3 unsaturated mayonnaise
2 ounces smoked wild-caught salmon, without sugar or preservatives
1 teaspoon capers
juice of ¼ lemon
salt and pepper to taste

Rinse the lettuce with purified water. Take 2 leaves, and spread a very light layer of mayonnaise on each lettuce leaf. Lay slices of the salmon along the leaves. Place the capers on top of the salmon, followed by the lemon juice. Salt and pepper to taste. Roll up the leaf and enjoy.

Yield: 2 rolls

PORTOBELLO SAUTÉ

Give your endocrine system a boost with this recipe, which is particularly delicious when served with quinoa or brown rice. Make sure to soak all the fresh vegetables thoroughly, as discussed, if they're not organic. If they're organic, rinse them with purified water.

3 tablespoons extra virgin olive oil
2 garlic cloves, peeled
2 Portobello mushrooms, sliced
1 red pepper, seeded and finely sliced
2 plum tomatoes, seeded and quartered
1 scallion, finely chopped
1 jar artichoke hearts (packed in water), quartered
4 tablespoons organic balsamic vinegar
sprinkle cayenne pepper
basil

In a pan, warm the olive oil on low heat for a few minutes. Be careful not to overheat or burn. Sauté the garlic for 2 minutes; add the mushrooms, red pepper, and tomatoes and sauté for 10 minutes on low/medium heat, stirring occasionally; add the scallion, artichoke hearts, and balsamic vinegar; allow the mixture to cook for 5 to 8 more minutes, stirring occasionally. Sprinkle with cayenne pepper. Garnish with basil leaves and serve.

Yield: 2 servings

ZUCCHINI SPLIT PEA SOUP

$\frac{1}{2}$ onion, chopped
1 to 2 cloves garlic, minced
$\frac{3}{4}$ cup green split peas
1 bay leaf
6 cups vegetable stock
6 cups diced zucchini
2 tablespoons mixed chopped herbs: fresh basil, thyme, and so on
2 teaspoons tamari
$\frac{1}{2}$ pound spinach or other greens
$\frac{1}{4}$ cup chopped parsley
1 small lemon, sliced thin

Place the onion, garlic, split peas, and bay leaf in a saucepan with 4 cups of stock. Bring to a boil, then cover and simmer for 40 minutes. Add the zucchini, the remaining stock, and the herbs. Cook for another 10 minutes. Remove the bay leaf. Puree the soup in a blender in batches. Return it to the soup pot. Add the tamari and adjust the herbs, if needed. Stir in the spinach or greens and the parsley and cook a few minutes more. Garnish each serving with a thin slice of lemon. This soup may also be served cold.

Yield: 4 to 6 servings

LENTIL VEGETABLE SOUP

2 cups lentils, washed
2 large carrots, chopped
8 cups water or vegetable stock
1 zucchini, chopped
1 onion, chopped
1 tablespoon parsley
2 cloves garlic, minced
$2\frac{1}{2}$ teaspoons salt
2 large celery ribs, chopped
1 slice fresh ginger
3 green onions, sliced

Combine the above ingredients in a large soup pot with a cover and bring to a boil. Reduce the heat and simmer, covered, for $1\frac{1}{2}$ to 2 hours. Before serving, top with sliced green onions.

Yield: 4 to 6 servings

FENNEL STICKS

Slice one large fennel bulb into sticks, similar to celery sticks. Serve it on a small plate after dinner to clear the palate before dessert. Fennel aids digestion, too.

BROCCOLI SALAD

1½ pounds fresh broccoli
salt water
3 hard-boiled eggs
2 tablespoons minced onions
⅛ cup natural unsaturated mayonnaise
cayenne pepper
tamari to taste

Boil the broccoli in salt water until tender. Chop the eggs finely and toss with the onions and broccoli. Mix in the mayonnaise. Add cayenne pepper and tamari to taste. Chill. This salad will be a favorite even with broccoli haters!

Yield: 3 to 4 servings

NOUILLES "SAUCE AUX NOIX"

½ pound rice or Jerusalem artichoke noodles
1 cup fresh parsley, chopped
1 teaspoon fresh basil
¼ teaspoon salt or 1 teaspoon tamari
½ cup olive oil
⅛ teaspoon cayenne pepper
¼ cup chopped walnuts or pine nuts
3 cloves garlic, minced
2 tablespoons boiling water

Cook the noodles. Blend all the other ingredients with a fork or in a food processor or a blender. Pour the sauce on the hot drained noodles, toss, and serve. This dish can be frozen or kept for some days in the refrigerator.

Yield: 3 to 4 servings

MISO VEGETABLE TOPPING

1 to 2 cups diagonally sliced vegetables (cabbage is a good choice)
1 to 2 tablespoons extra virgin olive oil
1 tablespoon dark miso (or more to taste)
1 teaspoon agave syrup or agave sweetener

Sauté all the ingredients in a frying pan, stirring constantly, until the vegetables are evenly coated. Cool before serving and store refrigerated. Or make a double batch and add to it 4 cups of cooked brown rice. In this case, serve it hot, garnished with toasted sesame seeds.

Yield: 2 to 3 servings

SPECIAL SPROUT SPREAD

   1 cup alfalfa, cabbage, clover, or radish sprouts
   3 tablespoons olive oil
   1 to 2 tablespoons lemon juice
   ½ cup mung bean sprouts
   ½ cup sprouted wheat berries
   ⅛ teaspoon gomasio seasoning
   sea salt to taste

Grind the first 3 ingredients. Blend in the next 4 ingredients. Refrigerate until ready to serve. This is a good basic spread that can be made ahead of time and kept in the refrigerator up to a week. Add mashed tofu or more oil, and it can be used as a dip.

Yield: 2 to 3 servings

CASHEW GRAVY

Thick and rich, with a plain, homey taste, it's ideal for grain loaves, burgers, and vegetable loaves.

   1 teaspoon white miso
   6 tablespoons raw cashews
   1¼ to 1½ cups water
   1 tablespoon arrowroot
   lemon juice to taste

Grind the nuts to a powder in a blender or a processor. Gradually blend in 1¼ cups water to make a smooth milk.

Yield: 2 to 3 servings

GINGER ASPARAGUS SALAD

This is a very spicy warm salad made with steamed slivers of fresh asparagus and lots of ginger and garlic.

   1 pound asparagus, tough ends removed
   2 tablespoons tamari
   2 teaspoons extra virgin olive oil
   6 cloves garlic, minced
   1 tablespoon rice vinegar
   1-inch piece ginger root, unpeeled, grated

Ginger Asparagus Salad (continued)

1½ teaspoon hot Szechwan peppers, or cayenne
½ teaspoon agave syrup

Slice the asparagus into match sticks by cutting each stalk into 3-inch lengths, then slivering the lengths into thin strips with a sharp paring knife. Steam the asparagus for 5 minutes or until crisp-tender. Toss the warm asparagus with the remaining ingredients and serve at room temperature.

Yield: 4 servings

APRICOT SAUCE

2 cups apricot nectar (apricot juice in a jar)
½ cup dried unsulphured apricots, cut into small pieces

In a saucepan, combine the nectar and the apricots. Cover and simmer 20 to 25 minutes or until the apricots are tender. Chill.

Yield: 2 to 4 servings

TOMATO-ZUCCHINI SALAD WITH FOURTH OF JULY DRESSING

This is a salad to make when you take a basket of extra tomatoes and zucchini to a friend and find that she has a basket of them for you!

3 (6-inch) zucchini, sliced
1 small sweet onion, cut in thin rings, with skin left on
2 large ripe tomatoes, chopped coarsely

Combine the vegetables in a large glass or crockery bowl. Pour the dressing over the vegetables and toss. Serve immediately.

Yield: 4 servings

FOURTH OF JULY DRESSING

¼ cup red wine vinegar
2 teaspoons brown rice miso
2 tablespoons lemon juice
1 small clove garlic, crushed
2 teaspoons fresh basil
dash each of dry mustard, paprika, oregano
freshly ground pepper, no salt
⅔ cup olive oil

Mix the vinegar, miso, and lemon juice. Add the garlic, basil, and spices and mix or shake well. Add the oil and stir or shake until the dressing is well blended.

Yield: 4 servings

LEMON HERB DRESSING

1 tablespoon agave syrup
5 tablespoons fresh lemon juice
3 tablespoons apple cider vinegar
1 small clove garlic, crushed
1 teaspoon fresh basil
¼ teaspoon fresh oregano
fresh cayenne pepper
salt
⅔ cup safflower or very mild olive oil

Pour the agave syrup into the bottom of a medium-sized jar. Add the lemon juice and vinegar and stir until the agave syrup is dissolved. Add the garlic, seasonings, and oil. Cap the jar and shake well until all the ingredients are blended.

To use fresh herbs: substitute 2 medium-sized fresh basil leaves, finely chopped, for the dried basil. In place of dried oregano, add 2 large sprigs (about 1½ inches long) of summer savory, finely minced. Add 2 tablespoons of chopped chives. Make the fresh herb dressing about an hour ahead so that the flavors may blend. Fresh herbs are preferred for all cooking needs.

Yield: 4 servings

GAZPACHO

A Spanish salad you can drink!

1 small onion, chopped
1 bell pepper, as ripe as possible, chopped (not seeded)
1 large cucumber, chopped (reserve a few slices for garnish)
3 ripe tomatoes, about 1½ pounds, peeled and chopped*
2 cloves of garlic, chopped
¼ cup cider vinegar
2 teaspoons sweet paprika
2 tablespoons olive oil
⅛ teaspoon cayenne pepper

Blend all the ingredients to a smooth puree a little at a time, blending in the vinegar, paprika, and oil. Place the puree in a glass or ceramic bowl, and mix very well. Chill. Garnish with the cucumber slices and serve cold. Gazpacho is best when made a day in advance.

*Peel ripe tomatoes by dropping them in boiling water for 10 seconds. Drain. Rinse. Remove stem end and slip off the skin.

Yield: 4 servings

SALSA VERDE

This is an uncooked green salsa. If you can find fresh tomatillos, by all means use them for this salsa, but don't substitute American green tomatoes. The flavor will be quite different.

1 (13-oz.) jar Mexican green tomatoes (tomatillos)
¼ cup white onions, chopped
1 chili, roasted, peeled, and seeded
1 tablespoon olive oil
1 tablespoon white wine vinegar
1 teaspoon garlic, minced
¼ teaspoon sea salt
¼ teaspoon cayenne pepper

Combine the tomatoes, onions, and chili and puree in a blender. Combine with the remaining ingredients.

Yield: 1¾ cups

AVOCADO DRESSING

1 small sweet onion
1 medium clove garlic
1 very ripe avocado
⅓ cup healthful unsaturated, unsweetened mayonnaise
½ to 1 teaspoon chili powder
dash each of cayenne, basil, and oregano
1 teaspoon lemon juice
1 small ripe tomato, cut in quarters
ripe olives (for garnish)
corn chips

In a food processor equipped with a metal blade, process the onion and garlic for a few seconds just to get them started. Then add the avocado, which has been peeled and cut into quarters; the mayonnaise; and the seasonings. Process until smooth. Last, add the tomato quarters and process a few seconds until the tomato is incorporated. Pour most of the dressing over a salad and mix well. Garnish with the remaining dressing and ripe olives. Serve immediately with baked corn chips.

Yield: 4 servings

SUMMER SALAD

⅔ cup cooked rice (brown)
4 teaspoons green onion, minced
4 teaspoons bell pepper, minced

2 teaspoons parsley, minced
4 tablespoons jicama or turnip, raw and sliced
4 teaspoons celery, minced
2 radishes, sliced
2 tablespoons mayonnaise (to taste)
dash of tamari
1½ teaspoons lemon juice
pinch of cayenne
1 tablespoon light wine
½ small tomato, seeded and cut into strips

Combine all the ingredients and chill.

Yield: 3 to 4 servings

TOFU-MISO DIP OR FILLING

8 ounces tofu, well drained
2 tablespoons sesame butter
2 teaspoons miso (dark or light)
2 tablespoons celery, minced (optional)

Mash the tofu, then add the sesame butter and miso. Mix thoroughly and add the celery if desired.

Yield: 3 to 4 servings

NUTTY OR SEEDY MISO TOPPING

1 cup chopped nuts (or sunflower seeds)
4 tablespoons dark miso
3 tablespoons agave syrup
1 tablespoon water

Combine all the ingredients in a small skillet and bring to a boil, stirring constantly. Reduce the heat and simmer about 2 minutes until the mixture thickens. Cool before serving and store it refrigerated.

Variations: Omit the nuts or use nut butter instead of nuts (reduce the amount to ⅓ cup). Add mustard, vinegar, lemon juice, minced garlic, or grated onion to taste.

Yield: 3 to 4 servings

ZUCCHINI AND YOGURT DIP

1 pound fresh zucchini
1 cup yogurt
2 cloves garlic, crushed
½ cup tahini

Zucchini and Yogurt Dip (continued)

2 tablespoons lemon juice
1 teaspoon salt
½ teaspoon pepper
2 tablespoons fresh parsley, finely chopped

Bake the zucchini in the oven until they become soft; then peel and mash them. Add the remaining ingredients (except the parsley) and mix thoroughly. Place the dip on a serving platter and chill. Decorate with the parsley just before serving.

Yield: 3 to 4 servings

TAHINI-MISO SPREAD

1 tablespoon lemon juice
½ cup tahini
¼ cup water
1 tablespoon miso (or more to taste)
2 tablespoons parsley, finely chopped
2 tablespoons chives

Mix the lemon juice with the tahini, then slowly add the water, and mix well until smooth. Add the miso, parsley, and chives.

Yield: 3 to 4 servings

FINGERTIP MINI

4 thin circles of carrots
4 slices of broccoli stems, peeled
4 slices of cucumbers
4 slices of yellow summer squash
4 slices of radishes
1 cup alfalfa sprouts
½ cup buckwheat greens

Use toothpicks and alternate the slices to make a colorful appearance. Serve on alfalfa sprouts and buckwheat greens. Perfect for dipping!

Yield: 3 to 4 servings

CONFETTI RICE SALAD

⅓ cup sunflower seeds
1½ teaspoons celery seeds
⅔ cup watercress or parsley, minced
¼ cup red onion, minced
2 cups cooked brown rice or other grain

2 teaspoons lemon juice
¼ cup olive oil
3 tablespoons cider vinegar
⅛ teaspoon dry mustard
⅛ teaspoon paprika
pinch of salt

Toast the sunflower seeds by stirring them in a dry pan on medium heat for a few minutes until they start to give off a nice fragrance. Add the celery seeds and stir a bit until their fragrance just starts to come out. Remove the seeds from the pan at once. Mix the watercress, onion, seeds, rice, and lemon juice in a good-sized salad bowl. Mix the oil, vinegar, and seasonings well to make a dressing. Mix the dressing with the vegetable-rice mixture and let it sit in the refrigerator to marinate for half an hour before serving.

Yield: 3 to 4 servings

WHOLE MEAL SALAD WITH MISO SAUCE

3 cups cooked long grain brown rice
½ cup chopped green onions
¼ cup chopped parsley
⅜ teaspoon dry mustard
2 tablespoons minced garlic
¼ cup vinegar
⅛ cup lemon juice
¼ teaspoon salt
dash of cayenne pepper
¼ cup olive oil

Combine all the ingredients and let them marinate at room temperature for 1 hour. Then serve the marinated rice with the following salad and the miso sauce.

SALAD

1 cup mixed sprouts
½ green pepper, chopped
¼ cup Jerusalem artichoke, sliced
1 stalk celery, chopped
2 tomatoes, quartered
1 cup cooked potatoes, cold, cubed
1 large beet, steamed and shredded
1 cup green cabbage, shredded

Salad (continued)

Combine in layers all the ingredients, placing the marinated rice mixture on the bottom. Serve with Miso Sauce (see the following recipe).

MISO SAUCE

1½ tablespoons light miso
¾ cup olive oil
¼ cup each of tamari, vinegar, and water
1 teaspoon ginger, peeled, grated
3 tablespoons agave syrup

Combine the ingredients in a blender; serve over the salad. This dressing keeps for 2 months in the refrigerator.

Yield: 4 to 6 servings

FALAFEL SANDWICHES

1 cup dried garbanzo beans
2 cloves garlic, minced
2 tablespoons fresh parsley, minced
¼ teaspoon cumin
1 tablespoon sesame tahini
dash of cayenne
2 tablespoons lemon juice
½ teaspoon salt
fine dry whole wheat bread crumbs, about ½ cup

Soak the garbanzo beans overnight. Sprout them for 3 or 4 days until the sprouts are about ½-inch long. In a food processor or a blender, grind together the beans, garlic, parsley, cumin, tahini, cayenne, lemon juice, and salt. Form balls about 1 inch in diameter. Roll them in the bread crumbs. Place them on a cookie sheet and bake at 350°F for 25 minutes, turning twice.

Yield: 3 to 4 servings

DRESSING

1 to 3 cloves garlic, finely minced
4 tablespoons lemon juice
3 tablespoons tahini (or enough to make a thick dressing)
pinch each of cayenne and cumin

Mix all the ingredients together thoroughly.

SANDWICHES

    1 small cucumber, finely chopped
    1 medium tomato, peeled, seeded, and chopped
    4 scallions, minced
    2 ounces alfalfa or mixed sprouts
    plain yogurt (optional)
    whole wheat pita bread

Mix the dressing with the cucumber, tomato, scallions, and alfalfa sprouts. Cut each pita in half. Place a spoonful of the vegetables in the pocket. Top with hot falafel balls. Lavish with yogurt or tahini miso dressing.

Yield: 2 sandwiches

HUMMUS

    1 cup garbanzos
    3 cups water
    3 cloves garlic, minced
    $\frac{1}{4}$ cup olive oil
    $\frac{1}{2}$ cup sesame tahini
    $\frac{1}{4}$ cup lemon juice
    $\frac{3}{4}$ teaspoon sea salt

Soak the garbanzos overnight, add garlic, and simmer for 2 to 3 hours until tender. If pressure cooking, use $2\frac{1}{2}$ cups water and cook for 1 hour. Combine the cooked garbanzos with the other ingredients and puree them all together in a blender or a food processor. This mixture can be thinned with water to make a dip.

Yield: 3 to 4 servings

SPINACH FETTUCINE WITH WHITE MUSHROOM SAUCE

    2 cups fresh soy milk or sugar-free almond milk
    16 medium-sized mushrooms
    3 to 5 cloves garlic, halved
    $1\frac{1}{2}$ tablespoons rice or whole wheat flour (rice flour gives a lighter texture)
    $\frac{1}{4}$ teaspoon sea salt
    pinch of nutmeg
    Italian pepper, crushed to taste
    1 pound cooked spinach fettucine

Combine the soy milk or almond milk, all the mushrooms, and the garlic in a heavy-bottomed saucepan. Place it over moderate heat and cook for 7 minutes, never allowing the soy or almond milk to boil. Stir often.

Spinach Fettucine with White Mushroom Sauce (continued)

Puree the mixture, along with the flour, in a blender or a food processor. Return the mixture to the saucepan and cook over low heat, stirring often until the sauce is slightly thickened, about 7 minutes. Just before it's done, add the salt, a pinch of nutmeg, and a pinch of crushed Italian red pepper. Serve over cooked spinach fettucine and enjoy!

Yield: 3 to 4 servings

DAIRY-FREE PASTA AL PESTO

2 cloves fresh garlic, minced
¼ cup walnuts or pine nuts
2 tablespoons unrefined olive oil
1 tablespoon light white miso
1 tablespoon fresh basil
½ cup spinach leaves, washed and dried
½ cup fresh parsley
1 pound natural spelt, rice, or quinoa or thin spinach pasta, boiled until tender and drained

In a blender or a food processor, mix together the garlic, nuts, and olive oil. Add the white miso and blend for 30 seconds. Add the basil, spinach, and parsley; blend briefly until the mixture has a pastelike consistency. Finally, toss it with hot pasta. *Note: For a change of pace, try buckwheat soba or rice noodles.*

Yield: 3 to 4 servings

CHUNKY EGGPLANT AND ROSEMARY SAUCE

2 medium onions, coarsely chopped
3 cloves garlic, chopped
2 stalks celery, chopped
2 to 3 tablespoons olive oil
2 tablespoons rosemary
1 large eggplant, diced with the skin on
4 cups fresh chopped tomatoes
1 cup stock (vegetable)
1 teaspoon cayenne pepper, or to taste
½ cup fresh chopped parsley

Chop the onions, garlic, and celery. Heat the oil in a large pot and sauté the vegetables for 5 minutes until golden. Sprinkle with the rosemary.

Dice the eggplant and add it to the pot. Stir briefly, then add the tomatoes with their juices (make sure they're not the pink plastic winter variety: these don't have enough flavor). Allow the sauce to come to a boil, then add the stock. Bring the sauce to a boil again and reduce it to a simmer, uncovered.

Put on water for the pasta. Add the cayenne pepper and half the parsley to the sauce and continue to simmer the sauce uncovered.

When the water has boiled, add the pasta, stirring until the strands have separated and the water is boiling madly. If the pasta is fresh, boil it only 2 to 3 minutes, until al dente, still slightly firm but not soft; if it's dried, it may need to boil up to 7 minutes. Test it occasionally. Drain and transfer the pasta to a warm bowl, pour the eggplant sauce on top, and toss. Serve it immediately, garnished with parsley and cayenne pepper.

Yield: 3 to 4 servings

RED SNAPPER EN PAPILOTTE

2 pounds red snapper fillets, or other fresh fillets
¼ cup melted butter or olive oil
2 tablespoons lemon juice
1 teaspoon tamari
1 teaspoon paprika
1 medium onion, sliced into rings
1 medium green pepper, sliced into rings
1 slice fresh ginger, grated

Brush the fillets with half the melted butter and sprinkle with the lemon juice, tamari, and paprika. Sauté the onion, green pepper, and ginger in the rest of the butter or olive oil in a large skillet for 5 minutes. Place the fillets on top of the vegetables, cover, and cook for 10 to 15 minutes, until the fish flakes with a fork.

Yield: 3 to 4 servings

MUSHROOM PÂTÉ

1 tablespoon olive oil
½ large onion, chopped
1½ cups mushrooms, minced
4 cloves garlic, minced
2 tablespoons sherry
1 pinch rosemary

Mushroom Pâté (continued)

½ teaspoon thyme
1 tablespoon tamari sauce
½ teaspoon salt
½ teaspoon basil, fresh, of course
2 scallions, chopped
2 stalks celery, minced
½ cup walnuts
½ cup bread crumbs, whole grain

Heat the oil in a skillet and add the onion. Sauté, stirring, until the onion is limp but not browned. Add the mushrooms, garlic, and sherry. Sauté 1 or 2 minutes until the mushrooms begin to juice. Stir in the rosemary, thyme, tamari, salt, and basil. Put the scallions, celery, walnuts, and bread crumbs into a food processor and combine them until minced. Add the mushroom mixture and blend. Put the mixture into a bowl and refrigerate for 2 hours. Spread it on bread and crackers, or hollow out a loaf of French bread and stuff it.

Yield: 3 to 4 servings

STUFFED ARTICHOKES

2 large artichokes

Wash and cut the tops off, removing about ½ inch. Put them in a pot of boiling water for 5 minutes, remove, and fill each artichoke with the following mixture:

finely grated cornbread crumbs or ¼ cup cornmeal
1 tablespoon fresh parsley
1 teaspoon fresh basil
½ teaspoon garlic powder
¼ teaspoon cayenne pepper
1 teaspoon gomasio seasoning

Slightly open each row of leaves on the artichokes and press a small amount of the mixture into each row. Put the artichokes back in the pot in 1 inch of water, and pour a little cold-pressed olive oil over each artichoke. Simmer until a leaf comes off easily, 15 to 20 minutes, on low-medium heat.

Yield: 2 servings

Stir-Fried Veggies Fu Yung

Use all fresh ingredients.

½ cup olive oil, cold pressed
1 slice fresh ginger
1 yellow squash, thinly sliced
1 green pepper, thinly sliced
1 Jerusalem artichoke (sunchoke), thinly sliced
1 green onion (scallion), thinly sliced
½ cup mushrooms, sliced
1 carrot, thinly sliced
1 stalk of celery, thinly sliced
4 spears broccoli, chopped
3 tablespoons tamari
3 cloves garlic, minced
2 teaspoons gomasio seasoning
½ cup mung bean sprouts
2 eggs, beaten (optional)

Heat the wok for 5 minutes with the olive oil in it. Add the next 11 ingredients. Add the gomasio seasoning. Keep turning the veggies for 8 minutes over medium-low heat. Add the sprouts; stir for 1 minute. Pour the eggs over the veggies. Lower the heat. Simmer until the eggs are cooked. Serve at once.

Yield: 2 servings

Sushi Platters

1 strip kombu (seaweed)
¼ cup rice vinegar (optional)
2 tablespoons barley-malt syrup
3 cups cooked brown rice
nori seaweed

Heat the kombu, vinegar, and barley-malt syrup until boiling. Lower the heat and simmer for 5 minutes. Remove the kombu and pour it over the rice; mix well.

Spread the rice on sheets of toasted nori seaweed. Place the filling of your choice in the center. For the filling, choose from sliced, toasted scallions; cooked spinach; sliced-lengthwise carrots; powdered or pressed horseradish; sliced avocado; pickled sliced ginger; and umeboshi plum paste. Roll the nori into a tight roll and let it sit to seal. Cut it carefully into circles.

Yield: 2 to 4 servings

ASPARAGUS POLONAISE

    2 tablespoons unrefined safflower seed oil
    ¼ cup chopped Fu
    2 pounds asparagus, cooked
    parsley, chopped, for garnish

In a small skillet, heat the oil and add the Fu crumbs. Sauté until
lightly browned. Sprinkle over the hot, freshly cooked asparagus
spears. Sprinkle the minced parsley over everything.

Yield: 4 servings

EGGPLANT CONTINENTAL

    1 eggplant
    1 onion, chopped fine
    1 green pepper, chopped fine
    1 tomato, chopped fine
    1 zucchini, thinly sliced
    1 clove garlic, minced
    4 tablespoons olive oil
    3 tablespoons red wine (optional)
    ½ tablespoon oregano
    ½ teaspoon gomasio seasoning
    ¼ teaspoon cayenne pepper
    2 tablespoons brown rice miso

Poke the eggplant with a fork a couple of times, then bake at 350°F
for 10 minutes. In the meantime, combine onion, green pepper,
tomato, zucchini, and garlic. Heat the olive oil in a large skillet and
sauté the mixture until the ingredients are limp and tender (do not
overcook). Peel the eggplant, chop it very fine, and add it to the skillet. Add the red wine (optional), oregano, gomasio, and cayenne pepper. Stir in the brown rice miso, then simmer the mixture for 40
minutes. Serve it hot or cold as a dip.

Yield: 3 to 4 servings

PASTA E FAGIOLI

    ¾ cup garbanzo beans
    ¾ cup navy beans
    1½ quarts water
    1 large onion, chopped
    2 carrots, thinly sliced
    2 stalks celery, chopped

1 large ripe tomato, chopped
2 bay leaves
1 teaspoon dried thyme
4 cloves fresh garlic, minced
2 tablespoons miso
salt, to taste
8 ounces fettucine, small elbows, or shell pasta (whole wheat, artichoke, or buckwheat)
extra virgin olive oil, optional
cayenne pepper, to taste
parsley, chopped (for garnish)

Combine the beans and wash them well. Place them in a large pot and cover with cold water. Allow the beans to soak 6 hours or overnight.

Drain the beans and rinse again; place them in a pot with 1½ quarts of water. Bring this to a boil, then cover the pot, reduce the heat, and cook at a simmer until the beans are almost done, about 2 hours. Add more water to keep the beans covered as they cook, if necessary.

Add the onion, carrots, celery, tomato, bay leaves, thyme, garlic, and miso and cook 30 minutes longer. Add salt to taste.

Cook the pasta separately in lightly salted water; drain it and combine with the beans and vegetables. Garnish each serving with a sprinkling of olive oil, if desired, and cayenne pepper and parsley.

Yield: 3 to 4 servings

CREOLE FISH FILLETS

¼ cup olive oil
¼ cup whole-wheat flour
1 cup hot water
1 pound fresh fish fillets, cut in 1-inch chunks
½ pound fresh tomatoes
½ cup green onions and tops, chopped
½ cup parsley, chopped
¼ cup green pepper, chopped
4 cloves garlic, minced
2 bay leaves
1½ teaspoons salt
½ teaspoon thyme
dash of cayenne pepper
1 lemon slice
cooked brown rice

Creole Fish Fillets (continued)

Prepare a roux by heating the oil in a large skillet and blending in the flour over medium heat. Stir it constantly until brown, being careful not to scorch it. Add the water gradually and cook the roux until it's thick and smooth. Add all the remaining ingredients except the rice. Cover and simmer for 15 minutes. Remove the bay leaves and serve the fish over hot rice.

Yield: 3 to 4 servings

RED SNAPPER VERA CRUZ

1 to 3 pounds red snapper or similar white fish, filleted
3 tablespoons fresh lime juice
6 tablespoons olive oil
1 medium onion, chopped
2 cloves garlic, minced
2 pounds tomatoes, skinned and chopped
1 bay leaf
½ teaspoon oregano
½ cup green olives, sliced (natural style)
salt to taste

To prepare the fish, prick it with a fork and cover it with lime juice. Let the fish sit for about 2 hours. Sprinkle it with 2 tablespoons of olive oil. Cover it with the following tomato sauce:

Heat 4 tablespoons of olive oil. Add the chopped onion and minced garlic. Sauté until soft. Add 2 pounds of chopped tomatoes and bay leaf, oregano, green olives, and salt to taste. Cook the sauce until some of the juices have evaporated.

Pour the tomato sauce over the fish and bake at 350°F for 10 to 12 minutes or until the fish flakes with a fork. Avoid overcooking or the fish will become tough and dry.

Yield: 3 to 4 servings

TEMPEH TURKEY WITH SAVORY GRAVY

2 pounds tempeh
1 cup oil, for frying

Savory Stock

1 to 2 tablespoons miso
1 tablespoon prepared mustard

½ sage leaf
¼ teaspoon rosemary
½ teaspoon thyme
3 cups water or stock
2 to 3 tablespoons kuzu, dissolved in ¼ cup water

Cut the tempeh into 2-inch triangles. Slice each triangle in half; 1 pound will yield 24 thin, bite-sized triangles. Heat the oil in a heavy pan; fry the tempeh until golden brown. Drain in a paper towel. Place the fried tempeh in a saucepan. Add the miso, mustard, sage, rosemary, and thyme to the water or stock and pour it over the tempeh. Bring the broth to a boil, lower the flame, and simmer at least ½ to 1 hour. Long, slow simmering results in tender, delicious tempeh.

When the tempeh is tender, dissolve the kuzu in water. Stir it into the broth with the tempeh. Continue to stir until the sauce thickens. Turn off the flame. Cover. Reheat slowly when ready to serve. Adjust the seasonings. Serve over wild rice stuffing.

Yield: 3 to 4 servings

TOFU BURRITOS

2 cups tofu, squeezed and shredded
2 cups hot salsa
2 cups black beans, cooked
1 cup seitan, minced
8 whole-wheat flour tortillas (warmed by wrapping in a tea towel and placing in a steamer or the oven)
1 cup radish sprouts
½ cup tomatoes, chopped

Place the tofu in a bowl with 1 cup of the salsa. Let this mixture marinate at room temperature for 30 minutes. Meanwhile, heat the beans in a saucepan. Mince the seitan to the consistency of chopped meat. To assemble the burritos, place a large spoonful of the tofu-salsa mixture in the lower half of the tortilla. Layer the beans, then the seitan, sprouts, tomato, and more salsa over the tofu. Roll the burrito away from you, folding in the two sides and tucking the top edge under as you roll. Bake on a nonstick surface for 10 to 15 minutes, then serve. Add more salsa if desired, hot stuff!

Yield: 4 servings

Gingery Miso Broth with Carrot Flowers

2 small strips kombu (sea vegetable)
3 to 4 shiitake mushrooms
2 quarts stock or water
2 teaspoons fresh ginger, peeled, grated
⅔ cup carrots for flowers
¼ cup miso (shir-o or kome)
½ cup water
3 scallions, sliced thin, for garnish

Rinse the kombu and the shiitake mushrooms; place in the stock or water. Add the ginger. Bring to a boil, lower the flame, and simmer for ½ hour. Remove the kombu and shiitake. Slice the kombu into long 1-inch-wide strips, then slice across the strips thinly. Cut the mushroom stems off the caps. Slice the mushroom caps thinly. Return the kombu and the shiitake mushrooms to the stock. Simmer gently. Cut the carrot flowers, then add them to the stock 10 minutes before serving, so that the carrots will cook slightly. Five minutes before serving, add the miso dissolved in ½ cup water. Garnish with sliced scallions.

Yield: 6 servings

Stuffed Mushroom Caps with Tofu

12 large mushrooms (caps and stems separated)
½ cup Fu crumbs
½ cup frozen tofu, thawed, squeezed dry, and mashed
2 tablespoons sherry or white wine
pinch each of sea salt and cayenne pepper
pinch of marjoram
1 tablespoon tamari sauce
3 tablespoons soy oil or olive oil
1 small onion, minced or grated
¼ cup chopped almonds or cashews
gomasio seasoning (garnish)

Mince the mushroom stems in a processor or by hand. Mix them together with the Fu crumbs and tofu. Add the sherry or wine, salt, cayenne, marjoram, and tamari and let the mixture marinate 15 minutes.

Place the mushroom caps facedown on an ungreased baking sheet. Preheat the broiler; lightly broil the mushroom caps until they're dry and wrinkled looking. Turn them over and broil them 30 seconds face up. Let them cool.

Heat the olive oil in a saucepan and sauté the onion until soft but not browned. Add the marinated tofu mixture and the nuts, and sauté 2 minutes. Mound this mixture into the mushroom caps, filling them as high as possible. Garnish with gomasio seasoning and broil until light brown. Serve them warm.

Yield: 2 servings

CARROT-ALMOND PÂTÉ

1½ cups almonds
2 cups grated carrots, chopped fine
2 tablespoons tamari
1 to 1½ cups water
3 tablespoons eggless mayonnaise (no saturated fats)

Blend the almonds into a nut meal (raw and roasted will give different tastes). Blend in the remaining ingredients until smooth, adding water to the desired thickness. Let the mixture sit in refrigerator about 30 minutes before serving. It can be used as a dip for, or served on top of, crackers and raw vegetable slices as a canape.

Yield: 2 to 3 servings

CANDIED YAMS

2 pounds yams
2 teaspoons extra virgin olive oil
1 to 2 teaspoons tamari
½ cup orange juice or water
2 to 3 tablespoons agave syrup

Peel the yams. Slice them into ¼- to ½-inch rounds. Line a baking or serving dish neatly with yams. Mix 1 teaspoon of the oil, the tamari, and the water or orange juice together; pour over the yams. Cover and bake at 375°F for 45 to 60 minutes. Mix the agave, orange juice or water, and remaining oil together; brush or pour this over the cooked yams, to give them a glazed look. Cover and keep warm.

Yield: 3 to 4 servings

KALE

Wash one bunch of kale greens well. If the leaves are large, slice them down the middle along the stalk; if small, leave them whole. Drop them in boiling water and cook uncovered for 5 to 10 minutes, depending on how you like them. Drain and serve.

WATERCRESS

Wash one bunch very well. Boil 3 cups of water in a skillet. Drop the watercress in boiling water for no more than 1 minute; then remove, chop, and place it in a small bowl. Add the following sauce: mix 3 tablespoons of almond butter and 3 tablespoons of light miso with distilled water to the desired consistency.

Yield: 3 or 4 servings

CRANBERRY KANTEN

1 quart apple juice
½ cup agar flakes, or one bar agar
2 apples, diced
1 orange peel
½ cup walnuts
2 cups cranberries
1 tablespoon kuzu
pinch of salt
¼ teaspoon cinnamon, optional
¼ cup agave syrup is optional for extra sweetness

"Kanten" is a name given to dishes thickened with agar. To make this one, pour the juice into a saucepan. Add the agar and stir; bring it to a low boil, then simmer for 20 minutes until the agar is completely dissolved. While the mixture is cooking, dice the apples, grate the orange peel, roast and chop the walnuts, and wash the cranberries.

When the kanten has cooked for 20 minutes, dissolve the kuzu in ¼ cup water; stir the kuzu into the kanten; continue to stir until the kuzu cooks and becomes clear. Now add the nuts, fruit, salt, cinnamon, and agave syrup. Simmer 2 to 3 minutes until the cranberries pop. Pour everything into a low, shallow serving dish. Allow it to cool to room temperature, then place it in the refrigerator. Serve it with the meal or as a dessert. This dish is best if made the day before.

Yield: 3 to 4 servings

MUSHROOM RISSOLES

These are individual, pyramid-shaped mushroom roasts to serve with cashew or brown gravy. This is a good choice for people who like to plan ahead, as the mixture should be chilled before shaping.

3 tablespoons canola oil
½ pound mushrooms, chopped (about 3 cups)
½ cup chopped scallions
2 stalks celery, minced
2 teaspoons gomasio seasoning
½ cup rice or almond milk
2 tablespoons soy flour
2 eggs, lightly beaten
1 teaspoon salt or tamari
1 cup cornmeal
½ cup combined walnuts and sunflower seeds, ground
½ cup wheat germ

Heat 2 tablespoons of oil in a skillet or a small saucepan and sauté the mushrooms, scallions, celery, and gomasio seasoning for 10 minutes. Gradually stir the milk into the soy flour and stir this mixture into the mushrooms. Cook, stirring, for 3 to 5 minutes until thickened. Remove it from the heat and cool slightly.

Add the eggs, salt, cornmeal, and nutmeal. Chill the mixture for several hours for easier shaping. When ready to cook, preheat the oven to 375°F. Form the mixture into 6 to 8 mounds. Dredge them with wheat germ. Place them on an oiled baking sheet and drizzle with the remaining tablespoon of oil. Bake them for 30 minutes.

Prepare a gravy while the rissoles bake, and spoon the gravy on top to serve. *Variation: For an egg-free version, increase the milk to 1 cup and the soy flour to* ¼ *cup.*

Yield: 2 to 3 servings

CABBAGE AU NATUREL

1 onion, sliced
¼ cup olive oil
½ cabbage, coarsely sliced
¼ cup apple cider vinegar
½ cup water
2 cloves garlic, pressed
¼ teaspoon thyme
½ teaspoon nutmeg
1½ teaspoons fresh dill weed

Sauté the onion and garlic in the oil; add the cabbage and the rest of the ingredients. Cook for 45 minutes over a low-medium flame or bake in the oven at 400°F for 45 minutes.

Yield: 3 to 4 servings

Spinach Mushroom Quiche

½ cup mushrooms
¼ cup black olives
2 tablespoons extra virgin olive oil
2½ cups mashed tofu
1½ cups almond milk
3 eggs
1 cup cooked spinach
¼ cup chives
½ teaspoon gomasio seasoning
¼ teaspoon cumin
½ teaspoon garlic powder
3 tablespoons light miso (mix in ¼ cup water)
whole-wheat crust, optional
sprinkle of paprika
½ cup green scallions, minced

You can make this with or without a crust. Sauté the mushrooms and olives in cold-pressed extra virgin olive oil. Combine the tofu and almond milk. Mix the eggs, spinach, chives, gomasio, cumin, garlic powder, and miso in a bowl and pour into the crust or directly into a well greased pie pan or a 10-inch glass baking dish.

Bake the crust at 450°F for 8 minutes, then put in the filling. Top with a sprinkle of paprika and minced scallions. Bake at 325°F for 40 minutes. Serve quiche hot or at room temperature. You may substitute the eggs with an additional 1½ cups of mashed tofu.

Yield: 4 servings

Roasted Sunflower and Pumpkin Seeds

1 cup sunflower seeds
1 cup pumpkin seeds
2 teaspoons tamari

On separate baking dishes, spread the seeds out evenly. Bake in 325°F oven. Stir occasionally to roast evenly. Check them after 10 minutes. When the seeds are golden, sprinkle them with tamari and stir to coat evenly. Allow them to cool. Store seeds in a jar.

Seeds or nuts can be roasted 3 to 4 days ahead, and are great to serve at a party. *Variation: Almonds, pecans, or filberts can be tamari-roasted, too.*

Yield: 2 cups

BIELER'S BROTH

equal amounts of:
celery
parsley
zucchini
string beans

Steam the veggies, then place them in a blender with pure water. You may puree or finely chop the mixture. You may add fresh garlic and a little tamari to taste. Heat gently; do not boil. Or put equal amounts of raw vegetables in a Vita-Mix and blend until the soup has a consistent texture.

Make this broth daily and eat or drink it two to three times a day. This broth will allow you to detoxify, while balancing your electrolytes.

CORIANDER AND GARLIC CRISP TEMPEH

Generations of Indonesian and American cooks have experimented with many natural seasonings to use with tempeh. Many agree that coriander and garlic are the most delicious.

½ teaspoon coriander, ground
1 clove garlic, crushed
½ cup water
2 teaspoons salt
6 ounces (170 gm) tempeh, cut into slices about 1-by-2-by-⅛-inch thick
oil for sautéing

Combine the first four ingredients in a bowl, mixing well. Dip the tempeh slices in quickly, then drain them briefly on absorbent (paper) toweling or a rack. Pat the surface lightly to absorb excess moisture. Heat the oil to 350°F (175°C) in a wok or a skillet. Slide in the tempeh and deep or shallow fry it for 3 to 4 minutes, or until crisp and golden brown. Drain it briefly on fresh paper toweling and serve immediately, either as is (as an hors d'oeuvre or a side dish), as an accompaniment for (brown) rice, or as an ingredient in other tempeh recipes.

Variations: Seasoned Crisp Tempeh—Prepare as above but omit the coriander and garlic.

Yield: 3 to 4 servings

GARBANZO BEAN CASSEROLE
    8 ounces cooked garbanzo beans
    6 ounces carrots or celery
    ½ cup green onions
    1 pound tomatoes
    2 ounces bell peppers
    ½ tablespoon vegetable seasoning
    ½ tablespoon paprika
    butter, to grease casserole dish
    ¼ to ½ cup cashew cream

Soak the beans overnight with three times as much water. The next morning rinse the beans, place them in a pot with twice as much water, cover, and bring to a boil. Reduce to a simmer for about 35 minutes. If you're using carrots, dice them into chunks and steam them for 15 minutes.

Dice the other vegetables and mix them with the garbanzo beans and seasonings. Place everything in a well-buttered casserole dish, cover, and bake at 325°F for 35 minutes. After 25 minutes, top with a layer of the cashew cream.

Yield: 3 to 4 servings

THERESA'S ITALIAN SPAGHETTI
    1 jar artichoke hearts, chopped
    4 or 5 cloves garlic, minced
    3 or 5 scallions, finely chopped
    1 teaspoon fresh basil, minced
    ¼ cup unrefined olive oil
    1 package spelt or brown rice pasta (use fettucine or linguini) *or* 1 package brown rice noodles *or* 1 package sesame noodles

For the noodles: Bring a large saucepan of distilled water to a medium boil. While the water is being heated, make the sauce.

In small saucepan, on low heat, sauté all the other ingredients (except the noodles) in the olive oil. Stir and cook for about 10 minutes, being careful not to burn the garlic.

When the water boils, add the noodles, and cook for 4 to 5 minutes, or according to the package directions. Drain the noodles and pour the sauce over them, quickly distributing it. You may add a pinch of cayenne pepper and/or sea salt if your diet allows. Serve the spaghetti with a tossed salad or steamed vegetables. Enjoy!

Yield: 3 to 4 servings

MISO SOUP WITH VEGETARIAN DASHI STOCK

Dashi Stock
3-inch piece kombu seaweed
2½ quarts water

Boil the kombu in water for 20 minutes. Strain out the kombu and use the remaining stock as follows (called dashi in the following recipe).

Miso Soup
6 cups dashi
½ cup red miso
½ cup white miso
1 cake tofu, cut into small squares
1 scallion, minced
tamari, to taste

Heat the dashi stock to boiling, then remove 1 cup and mix it with both types of miso until a smooth paste is formed. Return this to the soup pot. Turn off the heat. Drop in the tofu and cover the pot. Let it sit for 3 minutes. Pour soup into bowls, garnish with the scallion, and season with tamari.

Yield: 6 servings

CHILI SANS CARNE

¼ cup olive oil
1 medium onion, chopped
1 large green pepper, chopped
4 cloves garlic, sliced
1 teaspoon each salt and chili powder
½ cup bulgur wheat
2 cups cooked kidney or pinto beans
2 cups chopped tomato
1 tablespoon tamari sauce
1 cup water

Heat the oil in a good-sized pot on medium heat. Sauté the onion for a few minutes; the pepper a minute more; the garlic, salt, and chili powder briefly; then add the bulgur and stir a minute more. Add the beans, tomato, tamari sauce, and water. Bring everything to a boil, then reduce the heat and simmer, covered, for at least 30 minutes, preferably longer, stirring occasionally. The chili freezes well, too.

Yield: 4 to 6 servings

SEAWEED DELUXE

¼ cup unrefined extra virgin olive oil
2 large onions, sliced thin
⅓ package hijiki seaweed (rinse quickly in bowl, then soak 20 minutes in
    distilled water until soft)
1 tablespoon miso, optional
2 tablespoons brown rice vinegar
2 teaspoons kuzu (arrowroot), optional

Heat the unrefined extra virgin olive oil in a wok or a skillet and sauté the onions until soft. Add the soaked seaweed, including the liquid. Add the miso and the brown rice vinegar, stirring the hijiki for 5 minutes. Put the cover on for 7 to 10 minutes, stir again for 2 minutes, and add the kuzu (arrowroot) to thicken. Serve with brown rice.

Variations: Sauté the onions with ¾ cup eggplant and/or ½ cup red bell pepper. Add ¼ cup sesame seeds. Then proceed as above.

Yield: 3 to 4 servings

SZECHUAN EGGPLANT

1 medium-sized eggplant (1½ pounds)
2 teaspoons salt
2 tablespoons extra virgin olive oil
3 to 4 large cloves garlic, minced
1 teaspoon ginger root, minced
2 to 3 scallions, chopped
¼ to ½ teaspoon crushed red pepper
dash of wine or brandy
2 teaspoons tamari

Peel and cut the eggplant into strips, 1-by-2½ inches. Sprinkle them lightly with salt and let them sit in a bowl for ½ hour.

Heat the oil in a wok. When it's very hot, add the garlic and ginger; stir fry for about 30 seconds. Add the scallions; cook 1 minute. Add the eggplant and red pepper, stir fry for 30 seconds, turn the heat down (low), and cover; cook for 15 minutes, stirring occasionally. The eggplant should be very tender, almost like a puree. Add the liquor and tamari and serve with brown rice.

Yield: 3 to 4 servings

Appendix A:
Hypothyroid Testing

Hypothyroidism: The Unsuspected Illness, by Broda Barnes, M.D., is an excellent book that has helped me improve the health of my hypothyroid patients. Dr. Barnes recommends that you take your morning temperature sampling for ten days in a row, not just for three. Menstruating women should start this ten-day BBT sampling on the third day of their cycle. It's best to use a basal thermometer, which is more accurate than a regular oral thermometer. Use a non-mercury thermometer, which is the most environmentally friendly type of thermometer. It's also more accurate than any digital electronic thermometer for this purpose.

Dr. Barnes also suggests that the thermometer be used under the arm, while the person is lying quietly in bed, with his or her arm comfortably at the side. The temperature is taken upon awakening, before rising out of bed.

Dr. Barnes ventures that this test is a check on the most basic function of the thyroid gland and its ability to regulate the body's metabolism and to control temperature. An average of ten days is a very useful indication, therefore, of overall thyroid status. In many people, it may well be more accurate than the blood tests. BBT testing, however, is not infallible.

Like any other test, it should never be used alone to diagnose or rule out a thyroid condition or to dictate therapy. Ten-day BBT testing is simply helpful information to be weighed wisely. I use BBT with every one of my patients who will agree to do it, and I recommend that other practitioners do the same. BBT would be a useful addition to many thyroid-management regimens.

In regard to testing your thyroid activity, here's is how to do it at home:

1. At night, shake down a thermometer to below 95 degrees. Put a pen and a piece of paper next to your bed for recording your temperature. The next morning, upon awakening, put the thermometer under your arm, with the bulb in the armpit and no clothing between it and your skin. Leave it there for 10 minutes (use a snooze alarm if you wake up to an electric alarm). Just drowse there for 10 minutes.

2. When the time is up, take out the thermometer and read it. Immediately write down the result. (On waking, most people are a little foggy and may forget the reading.) This reading is called your early morning basal body temperature. The normal range should be between 97.8 and 98.2. This reading taken under the armpit is somewhat lower and more accurate than readings taken by mouth. If you have a low-grade infection, this may read higher than your normal. If it's in that normal range, you should repeat the procedure every day for a week or so. If you're menstruating, also do it on the second and third day of your period. If it's below the normal range, you're probably hypothyroid, and if it's higher, you're probably hyperthyroid or have an infection.

Since you can't always rely on blood tests to accurately detect the cause of your illness, you owe it to yourself to get a hormone saliva test. If you decide, after taking the self-assessment tests and following the program in this book, that you want to see a holistic health practitioner for a Thyroid-Stimulating Hormone saliva test, check the Resource Guide to find one of my affiliates in your area.

Appendix B: Electromagnetic Energy and Stressors

Medical research has established that we are electromagnetic beings who send and receive information in the form of electromagnetic energy. For example, cardiologists have long documented that the heart generates the strongest electromagnetic field produced by the body, but new evidence shows that this cardiac energy may be exchanged when people make contact with caring intent.

In Robert O. Becker's book *The Body Electric* and my first book, *Transform Your Emotional DNA*, you can read more about how we are just like antennas that send and receive mental and emotional (information) frequencies or wavelengths.

Very simply, a frequency is the number of times an electromagnetic wave cycles per second; it is called hertz. You know those electrical outlets in your house? Their frequency is 60 cycles per second.

In addition to research by Robert O. Becker, an article by the National Foundation of Alternative Medicine shares the results of its investigations in the area of bioelectricity and electromagnetic fields. I have personally explored this subject for two decades in Europe and around the world. Let's take a look at some known facts. Clearly, bioelectricity occurs in cells, due to proteins that pump specific ions (e.g., sodium, potassium) across our cell membranes to form an electrical potential similar to that found in a battery.

Traditional medicine uses tests to verify our electrical health. One is an electrocardiogram (EKG), which records the electrical activity of the heart, shows abnormal rhythms (arrhythmias or dysrhythmias), and detects heart muscle damage.

Another medical test commonly used to test our electricity is the electroencephalogram (EEG), which detects abnormalities in the electrical activity of the brain. The energy fields that are picked up from the heart by an EKG, and those from the retina, the muscles, and the brain by an EEG, arise because of the electrical currents that flow as the cells carry out their activities. Studies show that proteins behave in a similar fashion to the semiconductors used in computers, to rapidly transfer bioelectrical signals to keep us healthy.

This field of study may be crucial in helping us understand stress and how to deal with it. Every inanimate and living structure has a certain natural or resonant frequency. I'm sure you've noticed that when you meet some people, you resonate immediately with them. You may feel that you're on the same wavelength. Your assumption is correct. Some people fall in love at first sight and really do live a happy life together. This means that they're vibrating at a similar frequency.

Have you ever known someone with a good vibe? When any two objects have similar natural frequencies, they can interact without touching; their vibrations become coupled and resonate like dancers in perfect step. A soprano singing a high note that coincides with the frequency of a goblet can shatter it into pieces. This occurs because of the resonance between the high note and the glass. The atoms in the glass vibrate so strongly that they can't hold together, and the goblet breaks. Here's another example. When you tune in a radio or a TV station, you're locating the station's frequency by detecting the specific signal through resonance.

You can easily determine whether something is a stressor in your life and to your body. When you fail to resonate with something, no matter what it is, you feel out of step, out of control, or perhaps even tired and fatigued. These symptoms tell you that it's a stressor.

Appendix C: Research into NeuroPhysical Reprogramming

The NeuroPhysical Reprogramming (NPR) protocol was tested at an independent neurologist's office on five patients using a 22-electrode EEG, along with full-spectrum biofeedback reading, four more EEG sites on the occipital lobe of the head, and EMG (muscle response) skin temperature and conductance (the ability of a material to conduct electricity).

The patients were fully clothed and comfortable. After they were connected to the electrodes, I stated out loud various "trigger words," such as *health*, *disease*, *wellness*, *sex*, *cancer*, *death*, *life*, *birth*, *children*, *divorce*, *marriage*, *money*, *career*, *success*, and *failure*. We then noted the brain and the nervous system responses on the EEG, EMG, and so on.

The next step involved repeating the procedure using the NeuroPhysical Reprogramming protocol and homeopathic Neuro-Emotional Remedies while the patient was still connected to the same equipment. (Neuro-Emotional Remedies are high-potency homeopathic remedies with drainage properties that eliminate emotional issues anchored by identities.)

Although topics identical to the "trigger words" were used, the delivery was different. The patient said the topics aloud, instead of my saying them. The reason for this is that kinesiological testing, a small but important part of the NPR protocol, results in a very poor accuracy rate if the patient does not make the statements. (If the doctor states it for the patient, the doctor is essentially testing him- or herself and not the patient.)

After each process was completed, the patient was again given the same questions that he or she had responded to before the NPR session. The testing indicated that the patient no longer contained the energy patterns that were visibly apparent thirty minutes earlier.

As part of the NPR protocol, I tested a reflex point (Meta Point— Governing Vessel #16), which is located in the center of the occipital lobe. After discovering the Meta Point in 1993, I learned that it leads to the part of the primal brain that stores fundamental belief systems and identities. These identities act as an anchor, making a disease difficult to cure or heal.

The printout of the EEG and the other testing registered identical responses, so that each test confirmed the next. The printout indicated exactly when the homeopathic remedies were introduced to the patient during the NeuroPhysical Reprogramming protocol. You could see a heightened response and then a release.

A printout of the entire testing clearly indicated the neurological changes that occurred from administering the remedies on one patient and not another. Whether the issue was related to disease or sexual abuse, the process appeared to work the same. All testing indicated that NPR testing and the responses from the EEG, EMG, and so on, were identical and that Neuro-Emotional Remedies visibly released energy patterns.

Also worth noting:

* In another research project, Kirlian photography was used to measure the energy field of an AIDS patient before and after an NPR session. The Kirlian photographs were published in my book *Transform Your Emotional DNA*.

* The results of the testing indicated that NeuroPhysical Reprogramming and Neuro-Emotional Remedies released core issues stemming from identities that can be a major cause of mental and physical illness.

* NeuroPhysical Reprogramming and Neuro-Emotional Remedies have been used with measurable success on thousands of patients. Testimonials are available.

Recommended Reading

Articles

Artemisinin
depts.washington.edu/bioe/artemisinin.shtml
www.annieappleseedproject.org/artemisinin.html
www.drlam.com/A3R_brief_in_doc_format/Artemisinin.cfm#3

Dale, Theresa, Ph.D., C.C.N., N.D.
"Stop Replacing Hormones, Rejuvenate Them: Five Element Healing
Your Hormone Choices."
www.wellnesscenter.net

Null, Gary, Ph.D., Carolyn Dean, M.D., N.D., Martin Feldman, M.D.,
Debora Rasio, M.D., and Dorothy Smith, Ph.D.
"Death by Medicine"
www.lef.org/magazine/mag2004/mar2004_awsi_death_01.htm

Psycho-Neuro-Immunology Information:

www.wellness.org.za/html/pni.html
www.templeton.org/humbleapproach/faith_factor/default.asp
www.the-scientist.com
raptor.slc.edu/~synapse/papers/pni.html

Research

ADD and ADHD
Benson, D. F. "The role of frontal dysfunction in attention deficit hyperactivity
  disorder." *Journal of Child Neurology* 6 (supp) (1991): S9–S12.
Blackwood, A. L. *Manual of Materia Medica, Therapeutics and Pharmacol-
  ogy*, Second Edition. Chicago: 1922.
Bradley, P. R. *British Herbal Compendium*, Volume 1. Bournemouth, England:
  British Herbal Medicine Association, 1992.
Chabot, R. J., H. Merkin, L. M. Wood, T. L. Davenport, and G. Serfontein.
  "Sensitivity and specificity of QEEG in children with attention deficit or spe-
  cific developmental learning disorders." *Clinical Electroencephalography*
  27, no. 1 (1996): 26–34.
Dewey, W. A. *Practical Homeopathic Therapeutics*, Third Edition. San Fran-
  cisco: 1934.
Duke, J. A. *CRC Handbook of Medicinal Herbs*. Boca Raton, Fla.: CRC Press,
  1989.

Dyme, I. Z., B. J. Sahakian, and B. E. Golinko, "Perseveration induced by methylphenidate (Ritalin) in children. A research note." *Journal of Child Psychology and Psychiatry* 28 (1989): 897–902.

Kolata, G. "Ethical questions spring up as use of Ritalin mushrooms." *San Diego Union Tribune*, May 18, 1996.

Mesulam, M. A. "Large-scale neurocognitive networks and distributed processing for attention, language, and memory." *Annals of Neurology* 28 (1990): 597–613.

Peiper, H., and R. L. Hoffman. "ADD: The Natural Approach." *Natural Foods Merchandiser* (September 1997).

Reckeweg, H. H. *Materia Medica Homeopathica Anthomotoxica: Volume 1*. Baden-Baden (translation of third German edition of 1983): n.p., n.d.

Sokol, M. S., M. Campbell, M. Goldstein, and A.M. Keiechman. "Attention deficit disorder with hyperactivity and the dopamine hypothesis: Case presentations with theorectical background." *Journal of the American Academy of Adolescent Psychiatry* 28 (1988): 897–902.

Suffin, S., and W. H. Emory. "Neurometric subgroups in attentional and affective disorders and their association with pharmacotherapeutic outcome." *Clinical Electroencephalography* 26, no. 21 (1995): 76–83.

Bone Health

AlkalizeForHealth, www.alkalizeforhealth.new/Lcalcium.htm.

De Jong, Z., M. Munneke, W. F. Lems, A. H. Zwinderman, H. M. Kroon, E. K. Pauwels, A. Jansen, K. H. Ronday, B. A. Dijkmans, F. C. Breedveld, T. P. Vliet Vlieland, and J. M. Haze. "Slowing of bone loss in patients with rheumatoid arthritis by long-term high-intensity exercise: Results of a randomized, controlled trial." *Arthritis Rheumatism* 50, no. 4 (2004): 1066–76.

Drinkwater, B., S. Grimston, D. Raab-Cullen, and C. Snow-Harter. "Osteoporosis and exercise. American College of Sports Medicine Position Stand." *Medical Science Sports Exercise* 27, no. 4 (1995): i–vii.

Franklin, B. (6th ed. editor). *ACSM's Guidelines for Exercise Testing and Prescription*. American College of Sports Medicine. New York: Lippincott, Williams & Wilkins, 2000.

Kai, M.C., M. Anderson, and E. M. Lau. "Exercise interventions: Defusing the world's osteoporosis time bomb." *Bulletin of the World Health Organization* 81, no. 11 (2003): 827–30.

Lao Tsu. *Tao Te Ching*. Oral reference from *qi gong* masters. (centuries B.C.E.)

Lobstein, D. "Physical activity's magic." *IEEE Potentials* 9, no. 2 (1990): 27–29.

———. "Physical fitness, endorphins, and emotional stability." *Chinese Journal of Sports Medicine* 7, no. 4 (1998): 229–231.

Murphy, N. M. and P. Carroll. "The effect of physical activity and its interaction with nutrition on bone health." *Proceedings of the Nutrition Society* 62, no. 4 (2003): 829–38.

Nieper, Hans A. "Mineral Transporters." biomedx.com/bones/page8.html.

Seguin, R. and M. E. Nelson. "The benefits of strength training for older adults."

American Journal of Preventative Medicine 25, no. 3 (suppl 2) (2003): 141–49.

Sentman, D. "Schumann Resonances." *Handbook of Atmospheric Electrodynamics.* (1995), Chapter 11, 267–95.

Wallace, L., M. Boxall, and N. Riddick. "Influencing exercise and diet to prevent osteoporosis: Lessons from three studies." *British Journal of Community Nursing* 9 (2004): 102–109.

Boron

Green, N. R. and A. A. Ferrando. "Plasma boron and the effects of boron supplementation in males." *Environmental Health Perspectives* 102 (suppl 7) (November 1994): 73–77.

Helliwell, T. R., S. A. Kelly, H. P. Walsh, L. Klenerman, J. Haines, R. Clark, and N. B. Roberts. "Elemental analysis of femoral bone from patients with fractured neck of femur or osteoarthrosis." *Bone* 18, no. 2 (February 1996): 151–57.

Hunt, C. D., J. L. Herbel, and F. H. Nielsen. "Metabolic responses of postmenopausal women to supplemental dietary boron and aluminum during usual and low magnesium intake: Boron, calcium, and magnesium absorption and retention and blood mineral concentrations." *American Journal of Clinical Nutrition* 65, no. 3 (March 1997): 803–13.

Hunt, C. D., T. R. Shuler, and L. M. Mullen. "Concentration of boron and other elements in human foods and personal-care products." *Journal of the American Diet Association* 91, no. 5 (May 1991): 558–68.

McCoy, H., M. A. Kenney, C. Montgomery, A. Irwin, L. Williams, and R. Orrell. "Relation of boron to the composition and mechanical properties of bone." *Environmental Health Perspective* 102 (suppl 7) (November 1994): 49–53.

Meacham, S. L., L. J. Taper, and S. L. Volpe. "Effects of boron supplementation on bone mineral density and dietary, blood, and urinary calcium, phosphorus, magnesium, and boron in female athletes." *Environmental Health Perspectives* 102 (suppl 7) (November 1994): 79–82.

Naghii, M. R., and S. Samman. "The effect of boron supplementation on its urinary excretion and selected cardiovascular risk factors in healthy male subjects." *Biological Trace Element Research* 56, no. 3 (March 1997): 273–86.

Newnham, R. E. "Essentiality of boron for healthy bones and joints." *Environmental Health Perspectives* 102 (suppl 7) (November 1997): 83–85.

Nielsen, F. H. "Biochemical and physiologic consequences of boron deprivation in humans." *Environmental Health Perspectives* 102 (suppl 7) (November 1994): 59–63.

———. "Studies on the relationship between boron and magnesium which possibly affects the formation and maintenance of bones." *Magnesium Trace Elements* 9, no. 2 (1990): 61–69.

Nielsen, F. H., C. D. Hunt, L. M. Mullen, and J. R. Hunt. "Effect of dietary boron on mineral, estrogen, and testosterone metabolism in postmenopausal women." *FASEB Journal* 1, no. 5 (November 1987): 394–97.

Penland, J. G. "Dietary boron, brain function, and cognitive performance." *Environmental Health Perspectives* 102 (suppl 7) (November 1994): 65–72.

Breast Cancer

www.breastcancer.org/tre_sys_hrt_howEstWrk.html
www.wellnesscenter.net

Hormones and Stress

De Quervain, D., et al. "Stress and glucocorticoids impair retrieval of long-term spatial memory." *Nature* 394 (1998): 787–90.

De Wied, D. "The neuropeptide story." *Frontiers in Neuroendocrinology* 18 (1997): 101–13.

Endroczi, E. *Recent Developments of Neurobiology in Hungary*, Volume 2, K. Lissak (ed.). Budapest: Akademia Kiado, 1969, 27–50.

Kopin, I. "Catecholamines, adrenal hormones, and stress." In Krieger and Hughes (eds.), *Neuroendocrinology*. Sunderland, Mass: Sinaver, 1980.

Levine, S. "Stress and behavior." *Scientific American* 224 (1971): 26–31.

Newcomer, J., et al. "Decreased memory performance in healthy humans induced by stress-level cortisol treatment." *Archives of General Psychiatry* 56 (6) (1999): 527–533.

Natural Progesterone Cream

O'Connor, Anahad. "Possible Peril Found in Menopause Cream." *New York Times*, March 30, 2004, D-8.

Saliva Hormone Testing

Ayers, J., D. L. Birenbaum, and K. M. Menon. "Luteal phase dysfunction in endometriosis: Elevated progesterone levels in peripheral and ovarian veins during the follicular phase." *Fertility Sterility* 47 (1987): 935–39.

Belsky, J. L., B. Cuello, L. W. Swanson, et al. "Cushing's syndrome due to ectopic production of corticotropin-releasing factor." *Journal of Clinical Endocrinology Metabolism* 60, no. 496 (1985).

Berthonneu, J., G. Tanguy, Y. Janssens, A. Guichard, P. Boyer, J. R. Zorn, and L. Cedard. "Salivary estradiol in spontaneous and stimulated menstrual cycles." *Human Reproduction* 4 (1989): 625–28.

Challis, J., D. Sloboda, S. Matthews, and A. Holloway. "Fetal hypothalamic-pituitary adrenal (HPA) development and activation as a determinant of the timing of birth, and of postnatal disease." *Endocrinology Research* 26, no. 4 (November 2000): 489–504.

Dallman, M. F., S. F. Akana, K. Levin, et al. "Corticosteroids and the control of function in the hypothalamo-pituitary-adrenal (HPA) axis." *Annals of the New York Academy of Sciences* 746, no. 22 (1994).

Danutra, V., A. Turkes, G. Read, D. Wilson, V. Griffiths, R. Jones, and K. Griffiths. "Progesterone concentrations in samples of saliva from adolescent girls living in Britain and Thailand, two countries where women are at widely differing risk of breast cancer." *Journal of Endocrinology* 121 (1998): 375–81.

Dye, L., and J. E. Blundell. "Menstrual cycle and appetite control: Implications for weight regulation." *Human Reproduction* 12, no. 6 (1997): 1142–51.

Findling, J. W., W. C. Engeland, and H. Raff. "The use of immunoradiometric assay for the measurement of ACTH in human plasma." *Trends in Endocrinological Metabolism* 1, no. 283 (1990).

Gold, P. W., D. L. Loriaux, A. Roy, et al. "Responses to corticotropin-releasing hormone in the hypercortisolism of depression and Cushing's disease." *New England Journal of Medicine* 314, no. 1329 (1986).

Hermus, A. R., G. F. Pieters, A. G. Smals, et al. "Transition from pituitary-dependent to adrenal-dependent Cushing's syndrome." *New England Journal of Medicine* 318, no. 966 (1988).

Hofman, L. F. "Human saliva as a diagnostic specimen." *Journal of Nutrition* 131, no. 5 (May 2001): 1621S–5S. Saliva Testing and Reference Laboratory, Inc., Seattle, WA 98104. PMID: 11340128 [PubMed—in process].

Kannan, C. R. "Diseases of the adrenal cortex." *Disease-a-Month* 34, no. 613 (1988).

Kaye, T. B., and L. Crapo. "The Cushing syndrome: An update on diagnostic tests." *Annals of Internal Medicine* 112, no. 434 (1990).

Keizer, H. "Exercise- and training-induced menstrual cycle irregularities (AMI)." *International Journal of Sports Medicine* 8 (suppl 3) (1986): 137–74.

Keizer, H., J. Poortman, and G. Bunnick. "Influence of physical exercise on sex steroid metabolism." *Journal of Applied Physiology* 48(1980): 765–69.

King, D. R., and E. E. Lack. "Adrenal cortical carcinoma: A clinical and pathologic study of 49 cases." *Cancer* 44, no. 239 (1979).

Lee, K. A., J. F. Shaver, E. C. Giblin, and N. F. Woods. "Sleep patterns related to menstrual cycle phase and premenstrual affective symptoms." *Sleep* 13, no. 5 (1990): 403–09.

Meikle, A.W., R. A. Daynes, and B. A. Araneo. "Adrenal androgen secretion and biologic effects." *Endocrinology Metabolism Clinic of North America* 20, no. 381 (1991).

Orth, D. N. "Corticotropin-releasing hormone in humans." *Endocrine Review* 13, no. 164 (1992).

Orth, D. N., W. J. Kovaks, and C. R. DeBold. "The adrenal cortex." In *William's Textbook of Endocrinology*, 8th Edition. J. D. Wilson and D. W. Foster, eds. (Philadelphia: W.B. Saunders, 1992), 489.

Pirke, K. M., U. Schweiger, R. Laessle, B. Dickhaut, M. Schweiger, and M. Waechtler. "Dieting influences the menstrual cycle: Vegetarian versus non-vegetarian diet." *Fertility, Sterility* 46 (1986): 1083.

Quinn, S. J., and G. H. Williams. "Regulation of aldosterone secretion." *Annual Review of Physiology* 50, no. 409 (1988).

Reznik, Y., V. Allali-Zerah, J. A. Chayvialle, et al. "Food-dependent Cushing's syndrome mediated by aberrant adrenal sensitivity to gastric inhibitory polypeptide." *New England Journal of Medicine* 327, no. 981 (1992).

Ronkainen, H., et al. "Physical exercise-induced changes and season-associated differences in the pituitary-ovarian function of runners and joggers." *Journal of Endocrinology and Metabolism* 60 (1985): 416.

Seeler, L. R. "Cushing's syndrome." *Cleveland Clinic Journal of Medicine* 55, no. 329 (1988).

Ulick S., J. Z. Wang, J. D. Blumenfeld, et al. "Cortisol inactivation overload: A mechanism of mineralocorticoid hypertension in the ectopic adrenocorticotropin syndrome." *Journal of Clinical Endocrinology and Metabolism* 74, no. 963 (1992).

Van Goozen, S. H., V. M. Weigant, E. Endert, F. A. Helmond, and N. E. Van de Poll. "Psychoendocrinological assessment of the menstrual cycle: The relationship between hormones, sexuality, and mood." *Archives of Sexual Behavior* 26, no. 4 (1997): 359–82.

Vining, R., R. McGinley, and R. Symons. "Hormones in saliva: Mode of entry and consequent implications for clinical interpretation." *Clinical Chemistry* 29 (1983): 1752–56.

Vuorento, T., O. Hovatta, H. Kurunmaki, K. Ratsula, and I. Huhtaneimi. "Measurements of salivary progesterone throughout the menstrual cycle in women suffering from unexplained infertility reveal high frequency of luteal phase defects." *Fertility, Sterility* 54 (1990): 211–16.

Vuorento, T. and I. Huhtaniemi. "Daily measurements of salivary progesterone during menstrual cycle in adolescent girls." *Fertility, Sterility* 58 (1992): 685–90.

Vuorento, T., A. Lahti, O. Hovatta, and I. Huhtaniemi. "Daily measurements of salivary progesterone reveal a high rate of anovulation in healthy students." *Scandinavian Journal of Clinical Laboratory Investigation* 49 (1989): 395–401.

Watabe, T., K. Tanaka, M. Kumagae, et al. "Role of endogenous arginine vasopressin in potentiating corticotropin-releasing hormone-stimulated corticotropin secretion in man." *Journal of Clinical Endocrinology and Metabolism* 66, no. 1132 (1988).

Wentz, A. "Cigarette smoking and fertility." *Fertility, Sterility* 46 (1986): 365.

Williams, G. H. "Guardian of the gate: Receptors, enzymes, and mineralocorticoid function" (editorial). *Journal of Clinical Endocrinology and Metabolism* 74, no. 961 (1992).

Wilson, D., A. Turkes, R. Jones, V. Danutra, G. Read, and K. Griffiths. "A comparison of menstrual cycle profiles of salivary progesterone in British and Thai adolescent girls." *European Journal of Cancer* 28A (1992): 1162–67.

Wingfield, M., C. O'Herlihy, M. Finn, D. Tallon, and P. Fottrell. "Follicular and luteal phase salivary progesterone profiles in women with endometriosis and infertility." *Gynecological Endocrinology* 8 (1994): 21–25.

Wong, Y., K. Mao, N. S. Panesar, E. P. Loong, A. M. Chang, and Z. J. Mi. "Salivary estradiol and progesterone during the normal ovulatory menstrual cycle in Chinese women." *European Journal of Obstetrics and Reproductive Biology* 34 (1990): 129–35.

Young, W. F., Jr., J. A. Carney, B. U. Musa, et al. "Familial Cushing's syndrome due to primary pigmented nodular adrenocortical disease: Reinvestigation 50 years later." *New England Journal of Medicine* 321, no. 1659 (1989).

Silica

Balch, James F., M.D., and Phyllis A. Balch, C.N.C. *Prescription for Nutritional Healing,* Second Edition (Vonore, Tenn.: Avery Publishing Group, 1997), 28.

Wallach, Joel D., and Ma Lan. *Rare Earths Forbidden Cures* (Bonita, Calif.: Double Happiness Publishing Co., 1995).

Resource Guide

Adobe Acrobat Reader

Some of the links I have provided may require your downloading Acrobat Reader. You can download it free of charge from this Web site link: www.adobe.com/products/acrobat/readstep2.html.

Amygdala Information

www.viewzone.com/amygdala/index4.html

Biofeedback Equipment

www.bio-medical.com
www.wilddevine.com

Biological Dentistry Information

American Academy for Biological Dentistry
P.O. Box 856
Carmel Valley, CA 93924
fax: 831-659-2417

Books

Health and the 7-Step Program

The Body Electric
Robert O. Becker
www.amazon.com
Explores the fascinating research that proves how the body generates electromagnetic energies that influence health and well-being.

Transform Your Emotional DNA
Theresa Dale, Ph.D., C.C.N., N.D.
www.wellnesscenter.net
A self-help book offering exercises to help you still the mind and understand the anatomy of illness.

Earl Mindell, Ph.D., R.Ph.
www.drearlmindell.com
The Web site of this world-renowned nutritional researcher and author contains a wealth of authoritative and up-to-date information on nutrition, nutritional supplements, and how to use them to enhance health.

Earl Mindell's Vitamin Bible for the 21st Century, by Earl Mindell (New York: Warner Books, 1999).
A user-friendly encyclopedia of vitamins and the evidence-based medicine that explains how and why they promote optimum health and nutrition.

Earl Mindell's New Herb Bible, by Earl Mindell (Palmer, Alaska: Fireside Books, 2000).
Everything you need to know about herbs; the science explaining why they remedy specific conditions. This easy-to-read book shows you how to use herbs to achieve radiant health.

Earl Mindell's Anti-Aging Bible, by Earl Mindell (Palmer, Alaska: Fireside Books, 1998).
This comprehensive book addresses how vitamins, minerals, and other

natural substances can help slow or prevent the effects of aging.

Homeopathy

You can purchase most homeopathic books at a low price from www.minimum.com.

Materia Medica with Repertory, by
   W. M. Boericke.
   ISBN 0-68576-567-9 or ISBN
   81-7021-003-8
Or, you can access Boericke's *Materia Medica* online at:
   homeoint.org/books/boericmm/
   index.htm.
And you can access Boericke's *Repertory* online at:
   homeoint.org/books4/boerirep/
   index.htm.

The Science of Homeopathy, by
   George Vithoulkas. ISBN
   0-80215-120-5.

Organon of Medicine by Samuel Hahnemann. ISBN 81-7021-085-2.
Or you can access this book online at:
   homeoint.org/books/hahorgan/
   index.htm.
For anyone who can read German, you can access this text written in its original language online at: homeoint.org/books4/organon/index.htm.

Kent's Repertory with Word Index,
   6th edition.

A Dictionary of Practical Materia Medica, by J. H. Clark. ISBN
   0-85032-139-5.
Or you can access this book online at:
   homeoint.org/clarke/index.htm.

Divided Legacy, Volume 3, by Harris Coulter. ISBN 0-91302-896-7.

California College of Natural Medicine

Entry Level and Professional Trainings
   (PT)

NeuroPhysical Reprogramming (PT)
849 Almar Ave., Suite C189
Santa Cruz, CA 95060
tel: 800-421-5027
www.cconm.com

Cosmetics

Pure Mineral Color Cosmetics
Iredale Mineral Cosmetics, Ltd.
tel: 800-817-5665
info@janeiredale.com
(To order, go to:
   www.janeiredale.com.)

Skin Care
Devita Natural Skin Care
Glendale, Arizona
tel: 602-547-9174
in health food stores

Youthful Essentials by Sun Country
   Naturals, Inc.
is available at
   www.youthfulessentials.com
tel: toll-free 1-877-916-1212 and at all
fine health food stores.

Nonie of Beverly Hills
Beverly Hills, CA
Available at health food stores nationwide.

Barefoot Botanicals
San Francisco, CA 94114
tel: 1-888-rosehip
www.barefoot-botanicals.com

Gabriele Skin Care
Available at health food stores everywhere.

EMF Information and Equipment

To detect microwaves from cell towers and cell phones:
Microalert by lessemf.com

To objectively measure EMFs in your home, office, or anywhere:
Triaxial ELF Magnetic Field Meter, model 4080
Battery operated
F. W. Bell
Orlando, FL
tel: 407-678-6900

Exercise Classes

Yoga: www.bikramyoga.com will help you find Bikram yoga classes in your area, as well as internationally.
See also www.ashtanga.com.

Pilates Reformer: Studio Classes
www.pilates.com

Exercise VHS Tapes and DVDs

Chow QiGong System (a great qi gong video)
To order, e-mail: eastwestqi@aol.com
East West Academy of Healing Arts
Eastwestqi.com

On the Ball with Leisa Hart: Abs Workout for Beginners (VHS and DVD)
Romana's Pilates: Powerhouse Mat Workout (VHS and DVD)
On the Ball with Lizbeth Garcia: Pilates Workout for Beginners (VHS and DVD)
Yoga for Urban Living with Himalaya Behl (VHS and DVD)
(To order, go to www.naturaljourneys.com.)

Eye Health

Pinhole glasses for myopia and hyperopia (farsightedness), presbyopia (diminished focusing range with age), and astigmatism.
www.myopia.org/pinholes.htm

Fruit and Vegetable Wash to Remove Pesticide Residues, Bacteria, and Parasites

Your local health food store most likely carries this, but here are some online sources.

Veggie Wash
www.citrusmagic.com/veggiewash.html

Clean Greens

www.gaiam.com

Graphics and Design

John Higley Design
tel: 541-482-8805

Green Drink

For an alkaline body, my favorite green drink is
Greens First (great tasting)
Code for Ordering: 1730
www.doctorsfornutrition.com/a/1730/

Health and Evidence-Based Medical Writing, Editing, and Research

Kyle Roderick
kyle4@mindspring.com

Homeopathic Hospitals in the United Kingdom

The Royal London Homeopathic Hospital
Great Ormond Street, London WC1N 3HR
tel: 0207-833-7276
www.rlhh.co.uk/index.php

Glasgow Homoeopathic Hospital
1053 Great Western Road
Glasgow, Scotland G12 0XQ
tel: 0141-211-1600

Bristol Homeopathic Hospital
Cotham Hill, Cotham
Bristol, England BS6 6JU

tel: 0117-973-1231
www.ubht.nhs.uk/homeopathy

Tunbridge Wells Homeopathic
   Hospital
Church Road, Tunbridge Wells
Kent, England TN1 1JU
tel: 01892-542-977

Department of Homeopathic Medicine
The Old Swan Health Centre, St.
   Oswald's Street
Liverpool, England L13 2BY
tel: 0151-228-6808

Homeopathic Remedies

The Wellness Center for Research and
   Education, Inc.
Theresa Dale's
   Five Element Saliva Test
   Homeopathic Hormone Revitaliza-
      tion Formulas
   Neuro-Emotional Remedies
   Meta-Wellness Home Study
      Program
   Gallbladder/Liver/Kidney Flush Kit
www.wellnesscenter.net
tel:
   retail: 800-928-9088
   health professionals:
   866-962-6484

Dr. Dale's Affiliate Health Providers
www.wellnesscenter.net

Homeopathy Overnight
www.homeopathyovernight.com

National Homeotherapeutics
Madison, WI
tel: 800-888-4066
Your local health food store and pharmacy sell a variety of homeopathic
remedies, but some potencies may be
unavailable.

Macrobiotic Centers

Kushi Institute
P.O. Box 7

Becket, MA 01223
tel: 1-800-975-8744 and
   413-623-8827
Web site: www.macrobiotics.org
programs@kushiinstitute.org
Go to this macrobiotic directory, and
you can locate a macrobiotic center in
your area.
www.macrobioticdirectory.com/links/
   pages/Continents/North_America/
   United_States/-Macrobiotic_Centers/

Mail Order Organic Food and Food Preparation Equipment

The following are sources of organic
foods and supplies:
Living Tree
   www.livingtreecommunity.com
   tel: 800-260-5534
Raw Foods & Books
   www.rawfoods.com
Diamond Organics
   www.diamondorganics.com
   tel: 888-ORGANIC
Sun Organic Farms
   www.sunorganicfarms.com
   tel: 888-269-9888
Daily Blessing Foods, Inc. (organic
   meats supplier)
   tel: 888-862-5785
Best raw coconut oil
   See Raw Foods & Books on this list
Vita-Mix
   www.vitamix.com
   tel: 800-848-2649
Juiceman juicer
   Available in major department
   stores.

Organic Consumers Association

www.organicconsumers.org/index.htm
Contains a wealth of information
regarding genetically engineered foods
and the campaign to stop their spread,
organic agriculture FAQs, and other
invaluable information on organic eating and living.

Organic Cotton Sheets, Towels, and Clothing for Men, Women, and Children

www.underthecanopy.com
(Organic fibers are a great alternative for people with allergies and chemical sensitivities.)

Raw Food Restaurants

Alaska
Enzyme Express
1330 East Huffman Road
Anchorage, AK 99515
tel: 907-345-2330

Arizona
The Tree of Life Cafe
771 Harshaw Road
Patagonia, AZ 85624
tel: 520-394-1589

California
Roxanne's
320 Magnolia Avenue
Larkspur, CA 94939
tel: 415-924-5004

Raw Energy Organic Juice Cafe
2050 Addison (between Shattuck and Milvia)
Berkeley, CA 94704
tel: 510-665-9464

Beverly Hills Juice Club
8382 Beverly Blvd.
Los Angeles, CA 90048
tel: 213-655-8300

Au Lac
16563 Brookhurst St. (at Heil)
Fountain Valley, CA 92708
tel: 714-418-0658

Inn of the Seventh Ray
128 Old Topanga Canyon Road
Topanga, CA 90290
tel: 310-455-1311

Florida
Dining in the Raw
800 Olivia St.
Key West, FL 33040
tel: 305-295-2600

Living Greens
205 McLeod Street
Merritt Island, FL 32953
tel: 321-454-2268

Suzanne's Vegetarian Bistro
7251 Biscayne Blvd.
Miami, FL 33138
tel: 305-758-5859

Georgia
Sprout Cafe Shinui Living Food Learning Center
1475 Holcomb Bridge Road, Suite 200
Roswell, GA 30076
tel: 770-992-9218

Hawaii
Raw Experience
42 Baldwin Ave.
Paia, HI 96779
tel: 808-579-9729

Idaho
Akasha Organics
Chapter One Bookstore
106 North Main
Ketchum, ID 83340
tel: 208-726-5425

Illinois
Karyn's Fresh Corner
3351 North Lincoln Avenue
Chicago, IL 60657
tel: 773-296-6990

Massachusetts
Organic Garden
294 Cabot Street
Beverly, MA 01915
tel: 978-922-0004

Minnesota
Ecopolitan
2409 Lyndale Avenue South
Minneapolis, MN 55405
tel: 612-87-GREEN (47336)

Nevada
Go Raw Cafe and Juice Bar
2910 Lakes Town Center
Las Vegas, NV 89117
tel: 702-254-5382

New York
Caravan of Dreams
405 East 6th Street
New York, NY 10009
tel: 212-254-1613

Quintessence
263 East 10th Street (between 1st Ave.
   and Ave. A)
New York, NY 10009
tel: 646-654-1823

Life Thyme
410 Sixth Avenue
New York, NY 10014
tel: 212-420-9099

Oregon
Well Springs Garden Cafe
2253 Highway 99
Jackson Hot Springs
Ashland, OR 97520-9657
tel: 541-488-6486

Pennsylvania
Arnold's Way
319 West Main St., Store # 4 Rear
Lansdale, PA 19446
tel: 215-361-0116

Switzerland
Restaurant Hiltl
Sihlstrasse 28
Zurich, ZH, 8001, Switzerland
e-mail: info@hiltl.vh
tel: 41-1-277-7000

Washington, D.C.
Delights of the Garden
2616 Georgia Ave., NW
Washington, DC 20011
tel/fax: 202-319-8747

West Virginia
Healthy Harvest
309 N. Court St.
Fayetteville, WV 25840
tel: 304-574-1788

Raw Food Web Sites

www.rawandjuicy.com
www.dyingtogetwell.com
www.thegardendiet.com
www.shazzie.com
www.harmonious-living.com
www.livingnutrition.com
www.healthfullivingintl.com
www.foodnsport.com
www.transformationinst.com
www.rawlife.com
www.matthewgrace.com
www.therawworld.com
www.Paulnison.com
www.therawworld.com
www.davidwolfe.com
www.rawvegan.com/faq_various2.
   html
www.living-foods.com
www.sunfood.net
www.tanglewoodwellnesscenter.
   com
www.justeatanapple.com
www.waldorfhomeschoolers.com
www.rawfoodnetwork.com
www.rawfoodsupport.com
www.fruitarian.com
www.waisays.com
www.rawandjuicy.com/
   messageboard.html

Index